Handbook of Diseases of the Breast

J M Dixon MD FRCS
Senior Lecturer,
University Department of Surgery,
Royal Infirmary, Edinburgh, UK

J R C Sainsbury MD FRCS
Consultant Surgeon,
Huddersfield Royal Infirmary,
Huddersfield, UK

With contributions by

George Masterton MD MRCPsych
Consultant Psychiatrist, Royal Infirmary, Edinburgh, UK

Rhiannon Pugh MBChB MRCPsych
Senior Registrar in Psychotherapy, Royal Edinburgh Hospital, Edinburgh, UK

Foreword by

Sir Patrick Forrest
Professor Emeritus and Honorary Fellow,
(Department of Surgery), University of Edinburgh, Edinburgh, UK

CHURCHILL LIVINGSTONE
EDINBURGH LONDON MADRID MELBOURNE NEW YORK AND TOKYO 1993

CHURCHILL LIVINGSTONE
Medical Division of Longman Group UK Limited

First published 1993

ISBN 0-443-04982-3

British Library Cataloguing in Publication Data
A catalogue record for this book is available from the British
Library

Library of Congress Cataloging in Publication Data is
available

Typset by Datix International Limited, Bungay, Suffolk
Printed in Great Britain at the University Press, Cambridge

Handbook of
Diseases of the Breast

To our families, friends and patients.

Contents

Colour plates

Foreword

The explosion of literature on the nature of breast disease, particularly breast cancer, with over 150 new published reports each month, makes it impossible for any one doctor to keep up-to-date with the literature. A difficulty which is not helped by the modern trend for large multi-author texts containing exhaustive reviews, only too often providing a source for reference, rather than coherent guidance as to the best approach. Small wonder then that doctors, other health professionals, students and patients are confused.

Michael Dixon and Richard Sainsbury have supplied a real need in writing a straightforward account of the practical issues affecting breast disorders. They have done so on a 'fast track', so that the guidelines in this small volume can be readily revised and kept up-to-date. As both authors are committed to the day-to-day management of patients in comprehensive breast units, their views and advice carry considerable authority.

The enthusiasm with which they and their publishers have tackled this project deserves congratulations and merits success.

1993   P.F.

Preface

As surgeons interested in breast disease, we have been frustrated by the lack of an up-to-date text dealing with the breast and the conditions which affect it. There have been recent developments in understanding, nomenclature and treatment, but these have been slow to reach major textbooks. It was our aim to produce a short didactic handbook of the breast and its diseases, setting out our current knowledge and management of patients, which would be suitable for medical students, doctors in training – physicians and surgeons, nurses working in breast units and general practitioners. Only you, as the reader, can determine if we have been successful.

The book has been written and produced within a 12-month period in an effort to ensure that it reflects current views on breast disease. It would not have been possible to do this without great efforts from our secretaries, Monica and Sue, and the support and flexibility of Churchill Livingstone, in particular Katia Chrysostomou and Tara Mistry. Psychological problems in patients with benign and malignant breast disease are clearly of great importance and we are grateful to Dr George Masterton and Dr Rhiannan Pugh who contributed chapter 10. JMD acknowledges the generous support of the Cancer Research Campaign. To ensure that the book was readable and covered appropriate topics, it was critically appraised by Dr John Harrison, a general practitioner from Hinckley, Leicester, and Mr Wyn Lewis, surgical registrar. Their contributions have been greatly appreciated.

We also thank Professor Sir Patrick Forrest for contributing Figure 5.4, which incorporates the most recent data on breast screening, and for agreeing to write the Foreword.

1993
J.M.D.
J.R.C.S.

Introduction

1. The normal breast and congenital abnormalities

THE NORMAL BREAST

Between the fifth and sixth week of human foetal development an ectodermal ridge, called 'the milk line', develops bilaterally and extends from the axilla to the groin (Fig. 1.1). Segments then coalesce into nests opposite the fifth intercostal space and in humans all but one of these nests usually disappear.

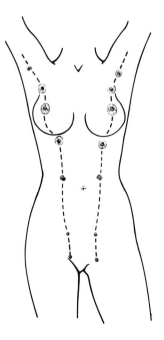

Fig. 1.1   The milk line or ridge.

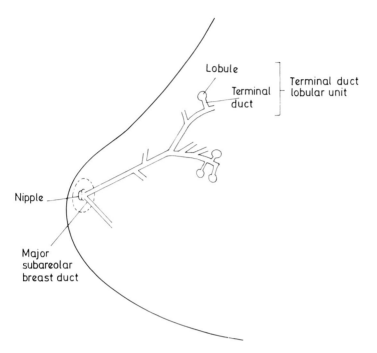

Fig. 1.2 The ductal and lobular system of the breast.

BREAST DEVELOPMENT

During puberty in girls, breasts increase in size, and within each breast ducts lengthen and the branching ductules at their ends develop buds which precede the development of breast lobules. At the same time connective tissue within the breast increases in volume.

THE ADULT BREAST

The breast lies between the second and sixth ribs on the vertical axis and between the sternal edge and the mid axillary line on the horizontal axis. Breast tissue also projects into the lower axilla as the axillary tail. The functional unit of the breast is the terminal duct lobular unit (Fig. 1.2) which drains into a series of branching ducts to form between 12 and 15 major ducts which open onto the nipple. The breast does not appear to be divided into clearly defined segments, as is often described, and the branching structure of the breast is not arranged in a true radial pattern, for instance all the breast tissue at 12 o'clock does not necessar-

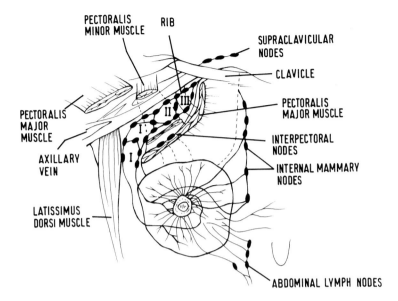

Fig. 1.3 Lymphatic drainage of the breast illustrating levels of axillary nodes.

ily drain into the major duct which opens at 12 o'clock on the nipple. The nipple and areola have certain distinctive features and the epithelium of the areola is more deeply pigmented than normal skin. At the edge of the areola there are prominent elevations formed by the openings of the ducts of Montgomery's glands which are large sebaceous glands. The subcutaneous tissues around the nipple contain smooth muscle which induces erection of the nipple.

BLOOD AND LYMPHATIC SUPPLY

The breast receives blood predominantly from perforating branches of the internal mammary artery and from branches of the lateral thoracic artery which enter through the axillary tail. The lymphatic drainage of the breast is important in relation to malignant disease. Lymph flow in the normal breast is from superficial to deep and the major drainage is then to the axilla and the internal mammary chain (Fig. 1.3). To a lesser extent, lymph also drains by intercostal routes to nodes adjacent to vertebra. The axillary nodes, which are found below the level of the axillary vein, can be divided into three groups in relation to the pectoralis minor muscle: level I lymph nodes lying lateral to the lateral border of the pectoralis minor muscle; level II nodes lying behind pectoralis

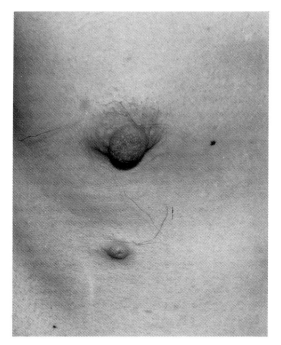

Fig. 1.4 Patient with an accessory nipple.

minor muscle; and level III nodes being located medial to the medial border of the pectoralis minor muscle (Fig. 1.3). Current evidence suggests that involvement of level II or III nodes is usually associated with level I involvement. There is an alternative route by which lymph can get to level III nodes without passing through nodes at level I and that is through lymph nodes on the undersurface of the pectoralis major muscle, the interpectoral nodes (Fig. 1.3).

CONGENITAL ABNORMALITIES

One or more of the other nests persists in 1–5% of people as a supernumerary or accessory nipple or, less frequently, as a supernumerary or accessory breast. The most common sites for accessory nipples are just below the normal breast in the milk line (Fig 1.4) and the most common sites for accessory breast tissue are the lower axilla (Fig. 1.5). Accessory nipples or breasts below the umbilicus are extremely uncommon. Supernumerary nipples and/or breasts rarely require treatment unless they are unsightly. Accessory breast tissue is subject to the same diseases found in normally placed breasts.

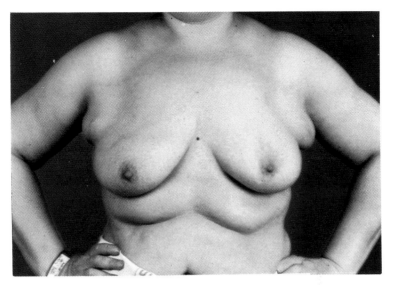

Fig. 1.5 Patient with bilateral axillary accessory breasts.

ABSENCE OF OR HYPOPLASIA OF THE BREAST

Introduction

One breast can be absent in isolation although it is more usual for this to be associated with pectoral muscle defects. Some degree of breast asymmetry is the norm rather than the exception, the left breast usually being larger than the right. Apart from developmental anomalies, tumours, surgery, radiation therapy and trauma can also all result in breast asymmetry. Abnormalities of the chest wall such as pectus excavatum and deformities of the thoracic spine may also result in symmetrical breasts appearing to be asymmetrical.

Treatment

True breast asymmetry can be treated by augmentation of the smaller breast, reducing or elevating the larger breast, or a combination of the two procedures.

2. Assessment and investigation of common symptoms

SYMPTOMS

An increasing number of women are consulting their general practitioner (GP) with breast symptoms. Not all such patients require referral to hospital. The important questions for the GP are:

- Is there a chance that cancer is present?
- If not, can I manage these symptoms myself?

The symptoms with which patients present to a breast clinic and their frequency are listed in Table 2.1. Painful, lumpy breasts are a common presenting symptom and a proportion of these could be appropriately managed in general practice. Only 10% of patients referred to hospital are ultimately shown to have breast cancer Guidelines for management:

- All patients with discrete lumps require referral to hospital for full assessment.
- Patients under the age of 40 with localized areas of tender nodularity should be re-examined following the next menstrual period. Those

Table 2.1 Presenting symptoms in patients attending a breast clinic expressed as a percentage (%)

Symptom	%
Breast lump	36
Painful lump or lumpiness	33
Pain alone	17.5
Nipple discharge	5
Nipple retraction	3
Strong family history of breast cancer	3
Breast distortion	1
Swelling/inflammation	1
Scaling nipple	0.5

in whom the nodularity persists require referral to hospital for further assessment.

- Young patients who present with tender, lumpy breasts who have no localized breast lesion but are symmetrically nodular can be reassured and do not require hospital assessment.
- Breast pain in the absence of a discrete palpable lesion can usually be managed adequately by the GP.
- Patients with nipple discharge, nipple retraction or distortion, a change in the skin contour, nipple eczema or patients presenting with a strong family history of breast cancer require referral to hospital.

METHODS OF ASSESSMENT

Introduction

Assessment of the breast starts with a careful history, proceeds to an examination and is supplemented by various imaging and biopsy techniques.

History

This includes details of age of menarche, age at which pregnancies occurred, age of menopause, menstrual regularity, usage of the contraceptive pill, family history and details of any medication. These can all be obtained by a simple questionnaire completed by the patient when waiting to be seen in the clinic. Details specific to the complaint are then sought.

The duration of the complaint is important — breast cancers grow slowly but cysts may appear overnight.

Examination

This starts with a detailed inspection in good light. The patient is examined with her arms by her side, above her head and pressing on her hips (Fig. 2.1). Skin dimpling or a change in contour should be sought. The causes of change in contour (in order of occurrence) include breast cancer, previous surgery, fat necrosis and sclerosing lesions. Deep seated lesions may only be evident in one of the three positions (Fig. 2.2). An assessment of the relative sizes (not often equal) and position of the breast can be made. Accessory nipples or breast tissue can be identified. The patient can be taught to do this in front of a mirror as part of becoming aware of her breasts and the range of normality (breast self examination is dealt with in chapter 5). The nipple

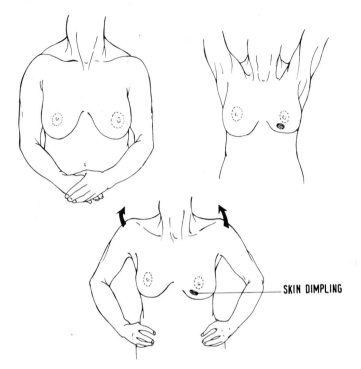

SKIN DIMPLING

Fig. 2.1   Clinical examination of the breast – positions in which breasts should be inspected.

is examined for any evidence of skin changes such as eczema or Paget's disease (Fig. 2.3).

The patient is then asked to lie flat and either place her arms above her head or on her hips. This spreads the breast against the chest wall and also allows access to the axillary tail which is otherwise covered by the patient's arm. Palpation commences with the hand held flat and aims to examine all the breast tissue rather than alighting on any dominant lesion (Fig. 2.4). Any lesion identified should then be further examined with the fingertips and assessed for deep fixation by tensing the pectoralis major by asking the patient to press on her hips. Once both breasts have been palpated the nodal areas are checked. The supraclavicular fossa and neck come first, followed by the axilla (which is often moist!). Examination of the axillary nodes is difficult and requires the co-operation of the patient. The weight of the arm needs to be taken by the examiner to remove tension in latissimus dorsi and pectoralis major muscles and palpation is then performed (Fig. 2.5). Nodes may easily be missed if the axilla contains a lot of fat and the correlation between clinical and pathological staging is poor.

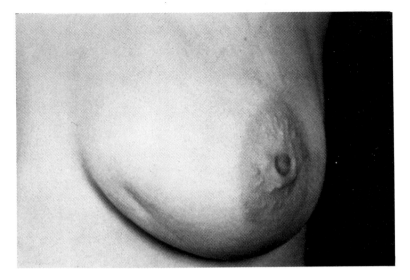

Fig. 2.2   All patients should be examined with arms by sides, above head and pressing on hips to look for changes in breast contour, as these may only be present in one of the three positions. This figure shows skin dimpling in the lower inner quadrant of the left breast associated with an underlying breast carcinoma.

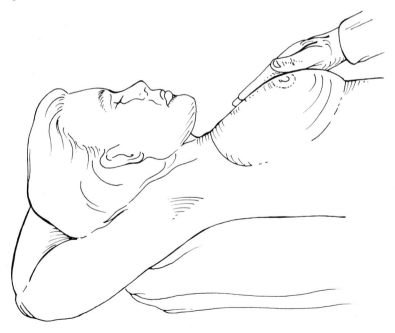

Fig. 2.4   Clinical examination of the breast – palpation.

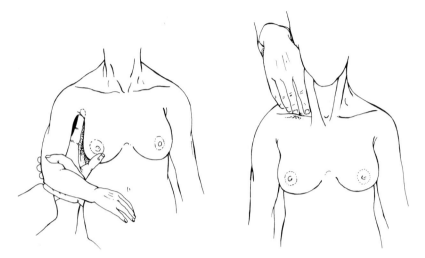

Fig. 2.5   Clinical examination of the breast – assessment of regional nodes.

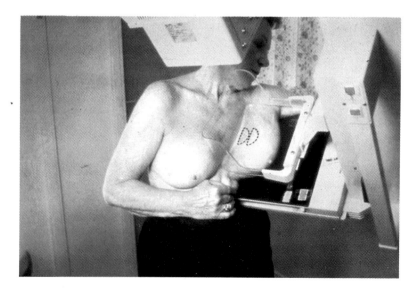

Fig. 2.6   Mammography being performed.

IMAGING TECHNIQUES

Mammography

The use of X-rays to obtain pictures of the breast was described in 1930 and is now the radiological investigation of choice. It requires that the breast be compressed between two plates while the exposure is made, which may be uncomfortable (Fig. 2.6). Single views of each breast may be taken obliquely, or two views obtained (oblique and craniocaudal). With modern film screens a dose of less than 1 mGY is standard. X-ray mammography has superseded xeromammography which, although more gentle for the patient, uses significantly higher radiation doses. Mammography allows the detection of distortion of normal architecture, masses (Fig. 2.7) and microcalcification (Fig. 2.8). The latter may be the only indication of early disease (such as ductal carcinoma in situ) and is the basis for the NHS Breast Screening Programme.

It is possible to carry out stereotactic cytology or to place a localization wire using an appropriate addition to the machine. The breast is held in a constant position and two pictures are taken at a standard angle from the vertical which allows the position of the lesion to be determined. By using needles of standard length the lesion can either be aspirated for cytological examination or marked with a hooked wire for later excision.

The breast is relatively radiodense below the age of 35 and higher exposures are needed to obtain good images. This, coupled with the relative infrequency of serious disease in this age group, means that mammography is rarely indicated in the under 35s. Figure 2.9 shows how the sensitivity of mammography varies with age.

Although some units allow open access mammography through GPs it is important that those who use the service are aware of the sensitivity and specificity of mammography. The current view would be that if the patient has a condition for which mammography is indicated then hospital referral is appropriate.

Ultrasound

This technique uses high-frequency sound waves which are beamed through the organ of interest. The reflections are detected and turned into images. Cysts show up as transparent objects and are easily detected. Benign lesions tend to have well demarcated edges, whilst the edge is often indistinct in cancers (Fig. 2.10). There is more subjectivity in the analysis of ultrasound and hard copy is generally disappointing. Some impalpable lesions detected on X-ray mammography can be seen on ultrasound and can be aspirated or marked using this technique.

Ultrasound may be used to examine the blood flow in tumours using the Doppler principle. False colours can be generated and the technique

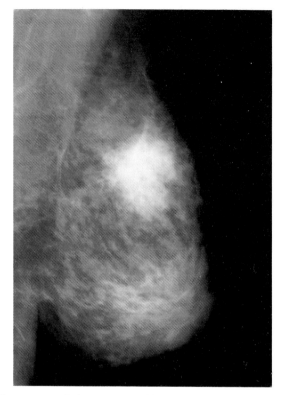

Fig. 2.7   Mammogram of a breast cancer with nodal metastases.

(colour Doppler) is being investigated in the diagnosis and management of both breast and axillary lesions.

One disadvantage is that the equipment is expensive and not widely available.

Other imaging tools

Computed tomography (CT)

This has proved disappointing for breast lesions although useful for metastatic breast cancer.

Magnetic resonance imaging

Early reports of this technique are promising and it potentially allows study of tumour metabolism. Further developments are occurring

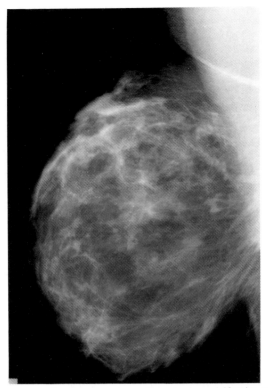

Fig. 2.8 Mammogram showing extensive malignant microcalcification which was impalpable.

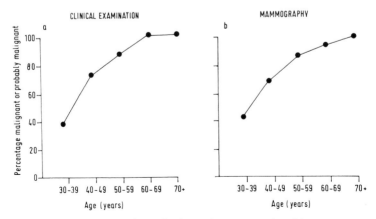

Fig. 2.9 Sensitivity of clinical examination and mammography with age.

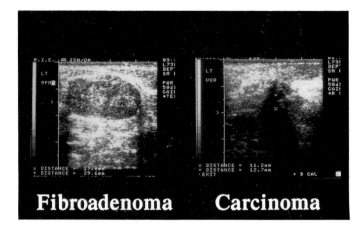

Fig. 2.10   Ultrasound of a fibroadenoma and a breast cancer.

rapidly although the equipment is expensive and limited in availability in the UK.

Thermography

Breast cancers may be warmer than surrounding breast tissue and techniques for evaluating this have been tried. Thermography using heat-sensitive paper has proved disappointing but microwave (10^{-15} M) radiation has been detected and attempts are being made to produce a brassiere with multiple detectors.

Radioisotope studies

These are mainly used to look for bony metastases. Ultrasound is more sensitive than radionucleotide scanning in assessing potential hepatic metastases. An injection of 600 MBq of ^{99m}Tc linked to methylene diphosphonate (MDP) is given and the patient placed under a gamma camera after 2–4 h. 'Hot spots' may be identified and often standard X-rays are needed to confirm if the lesions seen are metastatic or degenerative. The isotope detects areas of increased osteoclastic activity and false positives are therefore common.

Brain scanning can also be performed using radioisotopic techniques but CT is now generally preferred.

BIOPSY TECHNIQUES

Fine needle aspiration cytology (FNAC)

The ability to take material from a breast lesion without resorting to a formal biopsy and achieve a tissue diagnosis has been a great advance in the management of breast problems. It allows outpatient investigation with the potential to diagnose the majority of breast lesions at the patient's first visit.

FNAC requires skill in achieving adequate specimens and expertise in interpretation by the cytopathologist. In a few centres the cytologist takes the specimen, but in the majority the specimen is taken by the clinician and transported to the laboratory for analysis. To obtain reliable results care needs to be taken. A 21g (green) needle attached to a 10 or 20 ml syringe is used with or without a syringe holder. The latter may allow greater directional control whilst maintaining suction and increases the amount of material obtained, although some colleagues find it cumbersome and difficult to use. The needle is introduced into the lesion (this, in itself, gives useful information as the 'feel' of a carcinoma is very different from that of a fibroadenoma) and suction applied by withdrawing the plunger of the syringe (Fig. 2.11). Multiple passes through the lesion with changes in direction allow extensive sampling. The plunger is released prior to withdrawing the needle to keep the material in the needle. The sample obtained is then expressed onto microscope slides and gently smeared. The use of heparin to pre-wet the needle has been advocated by some but seems to be unnecessary. The slides are either air-dried or sprayed with a fixative (dependant on the cytologist's preference) and later stained. Stains used include the Giemsa, Papanicolaou or haematoxylin and eosin. A report can be given in about 15 min and some units provide an immediate reporting service. This can be useful if the initial sample is inadequate as repeat specimens can be taken at the first clinic visit. The major disadvantage is that it requires the time of a dedicated technician with access to a cytologist which in many centres is difficult to justify.

Reports are either given descriptively or on a numerical score (Table 2.2). Grade V smears are diagnostic of malignancy. There should be few, if any, false positive results in this category and many surgeons base definitive treatment on this report. Grade IV smears are highly suspicious for malignancy and usually 70–90% of these lesions will eventually turn out to be malignant. This category is useful as it allows the cytologist some leeway between a benign and a malignant call and is often used when only a few cells have been obtained or when the lesion is of unusual histology. Grade III is given if any atypical features are seen. The majority of these will still be benign although a proportion will be from carcinomas. Grade II reports indicate the material shows benign cells

Table 2.2 Reporting of fine needle aspiration cytology results

Grade	Result
AC0	No epithelial cells present
AC1	Scanty benign cells
AC2	Benign cells
AC3	Atypical cells present — may need a biopsy if clinically or radiologically suspicious
AC4	Highly suspicious of malignancy
AC5	Definitely malignant

with no atypical features. Sometimes specific diagnoses can be made. A fibroadenoma, for instance, may show many naked nuclei with branched chains of cells. Grade I indicates that only scanty material has been obtained and Grade 0 indicates that no epithelial cells have been obtained.

In some instances it is possible for the cytologist to classify the tumour and it is also possible to perform immunohistological studies on FNAC specimens to allow assessment of oestrogen receptor levels.

The combination of clinical examination, mammography and cytology is sometimes known as the triple approach. Combining all three allows a definite diagnosis to be made in the majority of patients presenting with a discrete breast lesion. Table 2.3 shows the effectiveness of each of these components.

Some GPs attempt aspiration of breast lumps. This allows them to diagnose those lesions which are cysts so giving the patients instant relief. As 1–3% of patients with cysts have breast cancer on clinical or mammographic examination at the time they present with their cyst, it is imperative that such patients are subsequently referred to a breast clinic for appropriate further assessment. Unfortunately a needle introduced by a GP into a lesion which is solid can result in haematoma formation and make subsequent assessment of this lesion more difficult. In some instances a haematoma which develops after fine needle aspiration can actually masquerade mammographically as a cancer. Routine aspiration of breast lumps by GPs is therefore not advised.

The suggested management of patients presenting with a defined symptom is given in figures 2.12–2.14. There will be overlap between these groups as patients may present with, for example, painful lumpy breasts.

Nipple cytology

Scrapings from the nipple or direct impressions of the nipple onto a clean glass slide have been advocated for the diagnosis of nipple lesions.

Table 2.3   Accuracy (%) of the different investigations in
diagnosing benign and malignant disease

	Clinical examination	US	Mammography	FNAC
% of cancers considered malignant or probably malignant (sensitivity)	88	85	88	95
% of lesions diagnosed malignant which are cancer (positive predictive value)	95	92	94	99.8
% of lesions diagnosed benign or normal which are benign (specificity)	91	88	90	95

US = ultrasound; FNAC = fine needle aspiration cytology

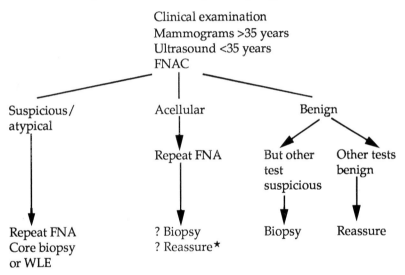

Fig. 2.12   Schematic diagram for investigation of a patient who presents with a
palpable breast lump. Patients with malignant cytology are not included.* Patients
with acellular cytology and lucent mammograms can be reassured.

The discharge (or aspirate) from a nipple can also be examined cytologi-
cally. We have found both disappointing and currently do not use them.

Core biopsy

The aim of this procedure is to remove a small core from the mass using
a cutting needle technique. A number of needles are available and some
can be combined with mechanical devices to make it possible to perform

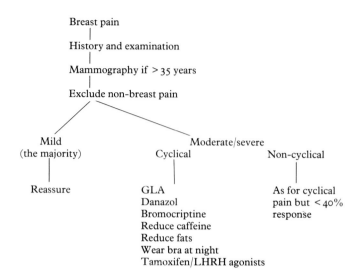

Fig. 2.13   Schematic diagram for investigation of a patient with breast pain.

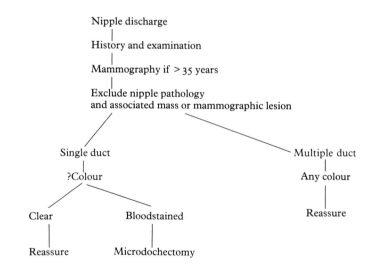

Fig. 2.14   Schematic diagram for investigation of a patient with nipple discharge.

the procedure with one hand, the other being available to fix the lesion being biopsied. While most patients tolerate needle biopsy it can cause considerable pain. It should only be used after FNAC and if a repeat FNAC is unlikely to give sufficient diagnostic information. After skin cleansing, local anaesthetic (1% lignocaine containing 1:200 000 adrenaline) is infiltrated into the skin, down to and around the lesion. This can make the mass more difficult to feel, but it ensures that the patient suffers as little pain as possible. Because of this, core biopsy is not recommended for lesions below 2 cm which can be easily excised under local anaesthesia. A small incision is strategically placed (11 or 15 blade) so that it can be easily removed at the time of definitive surgery, and so that the lesion can be approached at an angle of approximately 45° to the breast, to reduce the chance of damaging underlying structures in the chest or chest wall. The lesion is fixed between thumb and fingers of the left hand and the needle is introduced through the skin and breast until it abuts against the lesion. Fully mechanical biopsy guns are then fired and a core of tissue obtained. When using a needle alone or a needle in a hand-held 'gun', the open needle is moved forward into the lesion (Fig. 2.15b) and the sheath advanced to cut off a core of tissue (Fig. 2.15c). In hard lesions, advancement of the open needle is difficult and the whole needle should be advanced into the mass in the closed position (Fig. 2.15a) prior to pulling back the sheath which is subsequently advanced to obtain a tissue core. The biopsies are fixed in formalin, those which sink being more likely to give a diagnosis of malignancy than those which float. Frozen section reporting of core biopsies is advocated by some, but is not recommended. Bleeding is not usually a problem after core biopsy, particularly if adrenaline is added to the local anaesthetic solution, but it is appropriate to apply firm digital pressure over the lesion for several minutes. Finally the small skin incision is covered by an occlusive dressing. The result is usually available within 24–48 h. Because the procedure has a sensitivity of 80–90%, it is only of definitive value when a diagnosis of malignancy is obtained; a suspicious lesion with a benign core biopsy requires further investigation.

Open biopsy

If a diagnosis cannot be made by the combination of clinical examination, mammography and FNAC then an open biopsy may be necessary. Where there is a suspicion that the lesion may be malignant the excision should include a margin of normal breast tissue. The open biopsy may be performed as either an incisional or excisional procedure.

Incisional biopsy

This procedure should provide sufficient tissue to establish a diagnosis of invasive breast cancer and provide tissue for oestrogen receptor

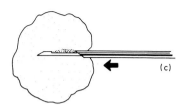

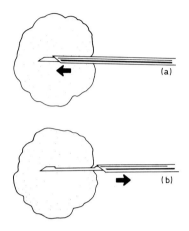

Fig. 2.15 Method of performing a core biopsy. The needle is advanced into the mass in the closed position (**a**); the sheath is withdrawn to allow the tumour to enter the notch of the needle (**b**); the sheath is advanced over the notch to cut off a portion of the tumour (**c**). The whole needle is then withdrawn.

analysis. This is not a therapeutic procedure and these patients will subsequently be treated either with primary systemic therapy, usually based on the oestrogen receptor content of the tumour, and/or radiotherapy. The incision over Langer's lines should be through normal skin, if necessary a small distance away from the tumour. The incision is best performed with a knife. After securing haemostasis, the wound is closed as for excisional biopsy.

Excisional biopsy

This technique aims to remove the palpable lesion with a minimal surrounding area of breast tissue and should be performed only if all investigations, including FNAC, suggest the lesion is benign. The skin incision should be curvilinear and follow Langer's lines (Fig. 2.16). Lesions within 5 cm of the areolar margin can be removed through a circumareolar incision which leaves an excellent cosmetic scar. Many apparently discrete lumps are nodular areas within the breast plate and these can be difficult to excise. For discrete lesions the fingers of the left hand are placed on the lesion and dissection with scissors (or if the tissue is dense, with a knife) is performed just beyond the tips of the fingers taking care to remove only a minimal margin of normal surrounding tissue. The size of the defect within the breast plate is an important determinant of the ultimate cosmetic result. If the lesion is grasped with tissue forceps, as is often suggested in operative texts, distortion of the lesion can make accurate excision difficult. Tissue forceps should only be applied when the lesion has been clearly defined and has been almost

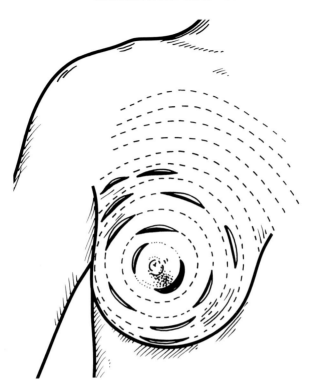

Fig. 2.16   Acceptable skin incisions for breast biopsy.

completely excised. Fibroadenomas usually lie within capsules and where this diagnosis is suggested by clinical examination, cytology and/or ultrasound, the lesion can be shelled out. Fibroadenomas are often attached to the breast by a small pedicle which is divided prior to removal (Fig. 2.17). Following excision the lesion should be fixed in formalin, unless it is considered to be suspicious at operation when it may be sent fresh. Haemostasis is secured with diathermy and drains should not be used. Suturing the defect in the breast frequently results in distortion and is not generally advocated. The wound should be closed in one or two layers with absorbable sutures – the lower layer being interrupted, deep, subcuticular sutures; and the superficial layer being a continuous, subcuticular suture. The use of interrupted sutures, clips or staples produce an inferior cosmetic result and their continued use cannot be defended.

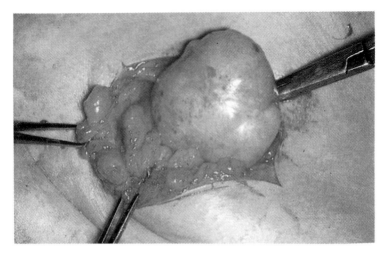

Fig. 2.17 A fibroadenoma being removed. (Reproduced with permission from Hughes et al 1989 Benign breast disorders and diseases of the breast. Balliere Tindall, London.)

Frozen sections

It used to be common to see on operating lists: 'frozen section ?proceed' (to mastectomy). This should now be obsolete as all patients should know what operation they are having when they leave the ward for the operating theatre (if not well before they are admitted for surgery). Hospitals and surgeons unable to provide a diagnosis prior to definitive treatment should not be undertaking this type of work. Frozen sections carry a higher false positive rate than FNAC and should not be used.

Frozen sections of the excision margins after a biopsy has been obtained are used by some surgeons to ensure completeness of the resection. This can result in considerable delay as the samples take time to process and be studied.

The use of frozen sections in the assessment of nodal status is also advocated by some. Four nodes are resected and sent for histology; if positive a further axillary procedure is performed.

Indications for biopsy of palpable lesions

The following are definite indications for biopsy:

1. When malignant cells are obtained from a lesion that is considered clinically and mammographically benign and either a mastectomy or a wide local excision and axillary node clearance is planned. The reason is that false positive results do occur with cytology, although

the positive predictive value of a malignant aspirate is over 99%. If a lesion is reported as malignant on cytology, and is clinically or mammographically malignant, a patient does not require further confirmation of the diagnosis prior to definitive surgery. In lesions over 2 cm a core biopsy is most appropriate; in masses below 2 cm or those between 2 and 4 cm where a core biopsy fails to confirm malignancy, then a wide local excision should be performed. For lesions over 4 cm an incisional biopsy is indicated.

2. When a lesion is considered suspicious of malignancy on clinical examination, mammography or cytology, it should be biopsied even when other investigations suggest it might be benign. For lesions over 4 cm a core biopsy may provide diagnostic information, but for the majority a wide local excision should be performed.

3. In cystic disease when a cyst contains evenly blood stained fluid, when a cyst persistently (greater than twice) and rapidly refills or where there is a persistent residual mass after aspiration (such a lesion must have been present on at least two occasions and have been investigated by FNAC) these patients should have the cyst and/or persistent mass excised. This is because cancers both intracystic and adjacent to cysts do occasionally occur. A wide excision is the surgical treatment of choice so that if the lesion is malignant the procedure is likely to be therapeutic.

4. A discrete breast lesion, even when considered to be benign on all modalities of investigation, should be removed by a simple excision biopsy if the patient requests removal. A lesion which is considered to be a fibroadenoma on all modalities of investigation can be 'shelled out'. Only a small minority, 10–20% of patients, who are informed their lesions are benign request excision.

   Some authors have suggested that all symptomatic patients over a certain age should have their lesions excised, based on the knowledge that as the age of the patient increases, so the chance it is malignant also increases (Fig. 2.18). This approach is illogical as numerous benign lesions, many of which are palpable are being identified during breast screening and are not being routinely excised. It is, however, useful to have guidelines for junior staff in breast clinics and it is not unreasonable to advise excisional biopsy of discrete breast masses in symptomatic women over the age of 40 unless there is unequivocal evidence that the lesion is benign (e.g. mammography showing a calcified fibroadenoma or lipoma).

5. Patients with large primary breast cancers, those with locally advanced breast cancers, and those who present with metastatic breast cancer, may require a core biopsy or an incisional biopsy to establish a diagnosis.

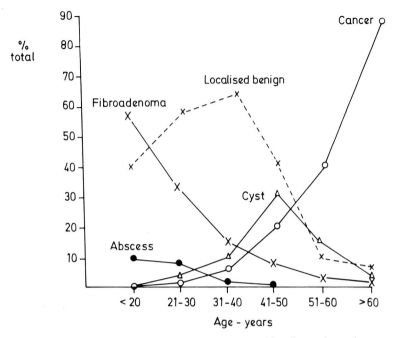

Fig. 2.18 Percentage of patients in 10-year age groups with a discrete breast lump who have common benign conditions and breast cancer.

It has been advocated that all patients undergoing surgical drainage of a breast abscess should have a biopsy of the abscess cavity. Performing aspiration in all masses which might be infective permits early identification and investigation by FNAC of those lesions which are solid, such as inflammatory carcinomas, and obviates the need for biopsy in this condition.

Assessment of patients with mammographically detected impalpable lesions

This group has become more frequent as the Screening Programme has got under way. One important distinction between these women and those presenting to the symptomatic breast clinic is that they are not 'patients'. They are essentially well (if worried) but extra reassurance is often necessary. In every case a definitive diagnosis and plan of action need to be formulated as uncertainty is a major component of worry.

Examination needs to be careful as subtle changes can be seen with even the smallest lesion. Localization of the abnormality with ultrasound or stereo X-rays may be needed, as may admission for a localization biopsy. The woman only becomes a patient when admission for diagnosis or treatment is needed. The number of women recalled for further X-rays at 6 months or a year needs minimizing.

Impalpable lesions

These are detected by mammography performed either during the investigation of symptomatic women or as part of routine breast screening. Patients with such lesions should be assessed by clinical examination, magnification mammography and ultrasound. Thereafter those which are truly impalpable and still considered suspicious of malignancy should have aspiration cytology using ultrasound or stereotactic guidance. This identifies some lesions as benign and these do not require further investigation (Fig. 2.20).

Technique for excision of impalpable lesions

The lesion is localized prior to operation by the radiologist using one of a number of techniques which may include skin marking, double dye injection or insertion of a hooked wire. The preferred method is the use of a hooked wire inserted using either ultrasound or stereotactic guidance. Following placement of the wire, true lateral and craniocaudal mammograms are taken and these films are discussed by the surgeon and radiologist prior to operation. From these two views the surgeon calculates where in the breast the lesion is likely to be situated and makes an incision along Langer's lines directly over this site (Fig. 2.16). The incision is deepened and dissection then proceeds in such a direction so the surgeon can identify the wire before it enters the lesion; for instance if the mammographic abnormality has been localized with the breast in the craniocaudal position, then dissection proceeds superiorly. Unless the lesion to be excised is widespread, as in some patients with microcalcification, the aim should be to perform an adequate excision. Once the wire is identified it is divided with sterile wire cutters, the proximal part of the wire being removed and tissue around the distal wire being grasped with tissue forceps. The wire itself should not be grasped as this may dislodge it. Using the mammograms as a guide, a block of tissue down to the pectoral fascia is excised (Fig. 2.19). This is then orientated with ligaclips. One way of doing this is to place one ligaclip on the anterior margin, two on the medial margin and three on the inferior margin, following which the specimen is X-rayed. Although it is suggested that specimen X-rays should be taken in a Faxitron, better quality specimen X-rays can be obtained using compression in a mammogram machine. Specimen X-rays must be inspected prior to

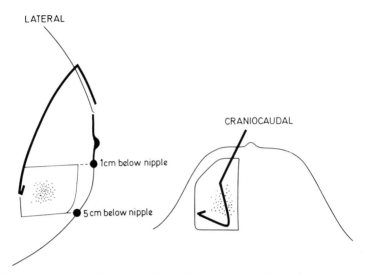

LATERAL

CRANIOCAUDAL

1cm below nipple

5 cm below nipple

Fig. 2.19 Diagrammatic representation of stereotactic-guided wide local excision of an area of microcalcifications.

wound closure to check the lesion has been excised. Orientation of the specimen has the advantage of allowing further tissue to be excised if the mammographic abnormality approaches any resection margin. Close co-operation between the surgeon and the pathologist is required to identify the nature of the lesion and the adequacy of excision margins. If the abnormality is not present in the first specimen, the surgeon should re-inspect the mammograms and further tissue should be excised and X-rayed. Failure to remove the lesion after three portions of tissue have been excised should lead to the termination of the procedure. Thereafter follow-up mammography is performed and, if appropriate, the patient should have a second localization procedure.

Indications for excision of impalpable lesions

The decision as to which lesions should be excised depends on the radiologist's degree of suspicion and the result of stereotactic FNAC (Fig. 2.20). Lesions which may require excision include:

1. a localized soft tissue mass lesion
2. an area of architectural distortion or parenchymal deformity (this includes stellate lesions)
3. clustered areas of microcalcification
4. a combination of the above features.

Recently a number of authors have questioned the value of stereotactic FNAC. It is the authors' view that as long as it is appreciated (by both clinician and patient) that the sensitivity of this procedure is less than that of FNAC of palpable lesions, then the advantage of avoiding many unnecessary biopsies and allowing definitive surgery combined with an axillary staging procedure at the first operation in the majority of patients with breast cancer far outweighs this disadvantage.

Type of anaesthetic for breast biopsy

All biopsy procedures can be performed under general or local anaesthesia; and the majority of simple excision biopsies should be performed under local anaesthesia. Although this is standard practice in the USA and in Scandinavia, many centres in the UK still advocate general anaesthesia for these operations which is difficult to defend, because local anaesthesia is acceptable to patients and more cost effective.

Intravenous sedation with midazolam makes the procedure more tolerable for anxious patients. Having palpated and identified the lesion to be removed, it should be marked on the skin either with an indelible marker or, if the skin incision is to be placed directly over the lesion, the skin can be scratched gently with the tip of a needle. This is important because once local anaesthetic has been infiltrated the lesion may be difficult to define. A 1% solution of lignocaine containing 1:200 000 adrenaline is infiltrated down to and around the lesion. During operation diathermy is utilized to secure haemostasis as for general anaesthesia.

It is current practice to perform the majority of excision biopsies under local anaesthesia, and the majority of wide local excisions and needle localization excisions under general anaesthesia. For these latter procedures it is important to be able to clearly define the margin between normal and abnormal breast, which is easier when the tissues are not swollen and distorted with local anaesthetic. Local anaesthesia is used in those patients who are unfit for general anaesthesia or where there is a specific patient preference.

Morbidity of breast biopsy

A breast biopsy performed for what is subsequently shown to be benign disease is not without morbidity. Immediate postoperative complications include haematoma formation and wound infection (in approximately 2% and 4% of patients, respectively). The incidence of these complications is not influenced by wound drainage or whether the operation is performed under local or general anaesthesia. Wound infection appears related to the nature of the underlying disease process and is most

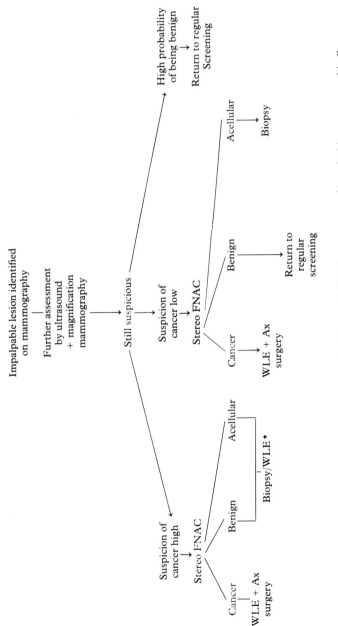

Fig. 2.20   Role of stereotactic fine needle aspiration cytology (stereo FNAC) in assessment of impalpable mammographically detected suspicious lesions. Ax = axillary, WLE = wide local excision, * extent of surgery dependent on degree of mammographic suspicion.

common following surgery for periductal mastitis, a condition from which both aerobic and anaerobic organisms have been isolated. A diagnosis of periductal mastitis can usually be made on the basis of the history and FNAC, and a biopsy is rarely indicated to establish the diagnosis. Operative procedures performed in patients with periductal mastitis should therefore be performed under antibiotic cover with Augmentin or a combination of cephradine and metronidazole.

Women undergoing breast biopsy suffer significant anxiety even when informed that the lesion is likely to be benign. This anxiety can be kept to a minimum by ensuring that the histological diagnosis is given to the patient as soon as it is available, which should certainly be within 10 days of the operative procedure. In the decade after breast biopsy for benign disease, 10% of patients develop a further breast mass at the biopsy site and a further 10% experience breast pain specifically related to the biopsy wound. A number of other women develop unsightly scars, either as a consequence of the postoperative complications of haematoma formation or wound infection, or because they produce hypertrophic or keloid scarring.

It has not been generally appreciated that breast biopsy is associated with such significant morbidity, as no study has followed up groups of women for long periods after these operations. Because of this potentially significant morbidity it is essential to keep the number of biopsies for benign disease to a minimum and it is suggested that the ratio of benign to malignant lesions excised in both symptomatic and screened women should be less than 1:1.

Non-malignant breast disease

3. Benign breast conditions

INTRODUCTION

Benign conditions of the breast are important because:

- They are more common than breast cancer and so account for the majority of attendances to a general practitioner and thus of hospital referrals.
- They can be difficult to differentiate from breast cancer.
- Incorrect diagnosis and inappropriate treatment of benign conditions is associated with significant morbidity.

Patients with benign breast conditions present with a lump, breast pain, nipple retraction or discharge, or are referred with a clinical or radiological abnormality found during breast screening. Most benign disorders arise on the basis of dynamic changes which occur in the breast through the three main periods of reproductive life: development (and early reproductive life), mature reproductive life and involution. The majority of benign conditions which affect the breast during these three periods can be considered as part of a spectrum from normal to overt disease. In between these extremes there are conditions which occur so frequently that they are most appropriately considered as aberrations rather than diseases (Table 3.1). The fact that there is a spectrum of change does not imply that these commonly occurring aberrations actually develop into disease.

ABERRATIONS OF NORMAL DEVELOPMENT AND INVOLUTION (ANDI)

Common conditions occurring during the stage of breast development which are best considered as aberrations of normal breast development include excessive breast enlargement during puberty (known as juvenile or virginal hypertrophy) and fibroadenoma. After the stage of breast development the breast undergoes periodic changes through successive

35

Table 3.1 Aberrations of normal development and involution

Age (years)	Normal process	Aberration
< 25	Breast development	
	lobular	Fibroadenoma
	stromal	Juvenile hypertrophy
25–40	Cyclical activity	Cyclical mastalgia
		Cyclical nodularity
		(diffuse or focal)
35–55	Involution	
	lobular	Macrocysts
	stromal	Sclerosing lesions
	ductal	Duct ectasia

menstrual cycles. Aberrations which occur during this period include breast pain and lumpiness or nodularity. In the past, specific terms such as fibrocystic disease and fibroadenosis have been used for painful lumpy breasts but these terms are no longer considered appropriate. The reason for this is that there is a very poor correlation between the presence of localized nodularity and pain and discomfort and what is going on at the pathological level. Breast involution starts in the fourth decade of life and includes: the development of small breast cysts (microcysts); focal areas of change in the normal epithelium lining breast ducts and lobules to sweat gland-type epithelium (apocrine change); an increase in the amount of fibrous tissue within the breast (fibrosis); an increase in the number of glandular elements within breast lobules (adenosis); and some increase in the number of cells lining the terminal duct lobular unit (minimal hyperplasia). Aberrations of this involutionary process include the formation of large breast cysts which present as palpable breast masses and excessive fibrosis which give rise to a series of abnormalities including the formation of radial scars and sclerosing lesions. Only when the epithelial proliferation within the breast lobules is excessive (moderate and florid hyperplasia) or is associated with atypical changes within the proliferating cells (atypical hyperplasia) are these changes considered as true disease.

JUVENILE HYPERTROPHY

Prepubertal breast enlargement in the absence of other sexual maturation is a common occurrence. Only if associated with other signs of sexual development is it an indication for investigation. Uncontrolled overgrowth of breast tissue occasionally occurs in adolescent girls whose breasts initially develop normally at puberty and then continue to grow often quite rapidly. This condition is called virginal or juvenile hypertrophy although it is not really hypertrophy; the histological features being an overgrowth of periductal connective tissue with proliferation of and an increase in branching of breast ducts without evidence of lobule formation. These appearances are no more than an exaggeration of the structure of a normally developing breast and this is why this condition is best considered an aberration of normal breast development. No endocrine abnormality can be detected in these girls.

Presentation

Patients present with a variety of symptoms: social embarrassment; pain; discomfort; inability to perform daily activities, such as regular exercise and walking down stairs; back and shoulder ache; and pain and discomfort directly under where the bra strap passes over the shoulder, where there is a characteristic indentation.

Treatment

Surgery significantly improves quality of life for many patients and should be more widely available. The aim of surgery is to reduce the size of the breast (reduction mammoplasty).

FIBROADENOMA

Although considered in most textbooks as benign neoplasms, fibroadenomas are best considered as aberrations of normal development because:

- Fibroadenomas develop from a whole lobule whereas neoplasms arise from a single cell.
- Fibroadenomatoid changes in lobules are common findings in the breasts of young women.
- Fibroadenomas show the same hormonal dependence as the remainder of the breast, for instance they lactate during pregnancy and involute during the perimenopausal period.

Incidence

Fibroadenomas account for approximately 12% of all palpable symptomatic breast masses. They are said to occur more frequently in Negro populations. The frequency with which they cause a breast lump in different ages in shown in Figure 2.18 (see page 26); they are a very common cause of a breast lump in women aged 15–25 years, but still account for 15% of all discrete lesions in women aged 30–40 years and are in fact a more frequent cause of a breast lump in this decade than cysts. Thereafter they are less common.

Classification

There are four separate entities of fibroadenoma: common fibroadenoma, giant fibroadenoma, juvenile fibroadenoma and phyllodes tumours. Fibroadenomas are characteristically classified by pathologists as intracanalicular or pericanalicular, but this histological distinction has no clinical relevance and the terminology can be abandoned. There is no universally accepted definition of a giant fibroadenoma but most consider that a fibroadenoma must measure over 5 cm in size to qualify for this definition. This type of fibroadenoma may or may not have a different behaviour to an ordinary fibroadenoma. The juvenile fibroadenoma occurs in adolescent girls and is rare. Most juvenile fibroadenomas undergo rapid growth and tend to be more cellular than ordinary fibroadenomas. These three entities are treated in an identical way.

Phyllodes tumours are distinct pathological entities and although they cannot always be differentiated from fibroadenomas clinically, their histology and behaviour are such that they should be classified as separate entities.

Presentation

Fibroadenomas usually present as a palpable breast lump, although they may be detected by screening. The majority are found in the upper, outer quadrant where most breast tissue is located. On examination they are usually well circumscribed, firm, mobile, discrete breast lumps and can occasionally be multiple or bilateral. A fibroadenoma is sometimes referred to as a 'breast mouse' because of its mobility within the breast tissue.

Diagnosis

Among the discrete breast masses thought clinically to be fibro-adenomas, 5% subsequently turn out to be carcinomas and clinical diagnosis may be incorrect in up to 50%. All discrete mobile lesions should therefore be fully investigated by mammography (if the patient is over the age of 35 years), ultrasonography (this is useful for women under the age of 35 and also for older patients with dense mammograms) and fine needle aspiration cytology (FNAC). Mammography can in some instances provide a definitive diagnosis of fibroadenoma when a well-defined lesion is seen containing characteristic coarse calcification. It is now accepted that it is possible to make a definitive diagnosis of a fibroadenoma by a combination of clinical examination, ultrasound (Fig. 2.10, see page 16) and FNAC.

Natural history

Current evidence suggests less than 5% of fibroadenomas increase in size, a number (approximately 20%) disappear and the remainder stay the same size but become clinically less distinct with time.

Management

It is routine practice in almost all units to remove those fibroadenomas over 4 cm in size. As fibroadenomas are benign and few increase in size, once a definitive diagnosis is established by a combination of clinical examination, ultrasonography and FNAC, a choice of treatments can be offered. The patient can be given the option of excision, performed under local or general anaesthetic, or observation which consists of a single follow-up ultrasound at 6 months to check the lesion has not increased in size. Some believe that observation is only appropriate in women under the age of 40 because of the possibility of missing a breast cancer in older women. The majority of women, given the option of observation or excision elect to keep their breast lumps. If access to good quality cytology and ultrasonography is not available, it is wise to excise all fibroadenomas to be certain that no malignant lesions are missed.

Phyllodes tumours exhibit a spectrum of behaviour ranging from benign to malignant, with a close correlation between the histological appearance and their subsequent behaviour. Only rarely do they metastasize and the main problem is of local recurrence. Treatment is by wide excision which in some instances means a mastectomy (which may be of the subcutaneous variety).

Relationship to breast carcinoma

Breast cancer is no more likely to develop in a fibroadenoma than in any other part of the breast.

MASTALGIA

Mastalgia or breast pain alone or in association with lumpiness is the most frequent reason for a breast-related consultation both in general practice and in specialist breast clinics.

It is best classified as non-breast mastalgia, cyclical and non-cyclical mastalgia.

NON-BREAST MASTALGIA

Conditions which have no association with either the breast or the chest wall sometimes present with apparent breast pain. A full history and careful clinical examination are required to demonstrate that the pain is arising from other organs. Non-breast mastalgia can be caused by angina, cholelithiasis, degenerative disorders such as cervical spondylosis, hiatus hernia, nerve entrapment syndromes such as in carpal tunnel or cervical rib, oesophageal lesions – particularly achalasia, pleurisy and pneumonia or pulmonary tuberculosis.

CYCLICAL MASTALGIA

Frequency

The exact incidence of cyclical mastalgia is not known but, when directly questioned, 66% of a group of working women and 70% of a screened population admitted to having had recent breast pain, with symptoms being severe in up to one-third. Breast pain is the main presenting symptom in about 50% of patients attending breast clinics. Classically women report that they have heightened awareness, discomfort, fullness and heaviness of their breasts during the 3–7 days which precede each menstrual period. During this period women often report that their breasts increase in size and that they develop areas of tender lumpiness. Following the commencement of menstrual flow these symptoms disappear. Some patients report extreme discomfort during these few days while others report pain and discomfort which last much longer than a few days and which can start within a few days of cessation of menstruation and continue until the next period. The frequency of mastalgia suggests that it should not be considered as a disease but is best considered as an aberration of normal cyclical changes within the reproductive years. The impact of mastalgia on quality of life is often underestimated by the medical profession. Mastalgia is very uncommon as a presenting feature of breast cancer.

Aetiology

Mastalgia shows many features which suggest that it has a hormonal basis, but no consistent hormonal abnormalities have been identified. Hormonal agents which improve mastalgia act at different sites on the hypothalamic–pituitary–ovarian–breast axis and this makes it likely that the aetiology of mastalgia is either multifactorial or that the final common pathway is at the breast cell level.

Water retention within the breast has been suggested as a cause of both mastalgia and the premenstrual tension syndrome because women report weight gain and breast and ankle swelling late in the menstrual cycle. Studies have shown that patients with mastalgia do not retain more water than women without this symptom. This information combined with the finding that diuretics are no more effective in mastalgia than placebo suggests that water retention is unlikely to be the cause of cyclical mastalgia.

A theory prevalent some years ago was that patients with mastalgia were more neurotic than other patients and that this manifested itself as a complaint of breast pain. This has now been shown conclusively to have no scientific foundation.

The role of essential fatty acids (EFAs)

The chance finding that there was a reduction in breast pain in women treated with evening primrose oil (EPO), which contains high levels of gamma linolenic acid (GLA), led to the investigation of the role of GLA and other EFAs in patients with mastalgia. EFAs must be provided regularly in the diet and have three major functions:

1. They are key determinants of cellular membrane flexibility and fluidity.

   In cellular membranes, EFAs are present as either free fatty acids, triglycerides or are esterified to phospholipids and cholesterol, and they compete with saturated fatty acids for incorporation into these membranes. EFAs confer the properties of flexibility and fluidity to membranes and thereby affect the activity of membrane-bound receptors. Hormone receptors, present within cellular membranes rich in saturated fatty acids, have a greater affinity for their respective hormones than those receptors found in membranes rich in polyunsaturated fatty acids. Therefore in an environment with a high saturated to polyunsaturated fatty acid ratio, increased receptor affinity and hormone potency will result in an exaggerated end organ response to normal circulating hormone levels.

2. They are precursors of biologically active metabolites.

   The metabolites of GLA are precursors of a wide range of short-lived biologically active molecules, which regulate many aspects of cellular activity, collectively known as the eicosanoids; prostaglandins, leukotrienes and other derivatives are produced locally as and when required and have a purely local effect after which they are eliminated. Prostaglandin E_1 (PGE_1), which is produced from EFAs, is known to be a second messenger for prolactin, and as prolactin levels rise, PGE_1 formation increases to switch off the peripheral effect of prolactin. Low levels of GLA and its metabolites therefore may result in a reduction of the levels of PGE_1 and lead to an exaggerated end organ response to prolactin.

The effects of GLA on membrane receptors and on eicosanoid and prostaglandin production might explain why normal levels of hormones produce exaggerated effects such as severe mastalgia.

3. EFAs have a role in the transport of cholesterol.

Cholesterol is transported to cells in low density lipoproteins (LDLs) and from cells to the liver in high density lipoproteins (HDLs). Women with mastalgia have been reported to have high levels of HDLs and low levels of LDLs in the absence of a difference in dietary fat intake.

Interestingly, hormonal drug treatments which improve symptoms of mastalgia influence plasma lipids, generally by producing a reduction in HDLs. The effect of GLA on plasma lipids is poorly described but it has been reported to reduce total cholesterol and to have variable effects on HDLs and LDLs. In view of the action of the recognized treatments for mastalgia on lipid metabolism, it is possible that the underlying aetiology of patients with mastalgia could be an abnormality in lipid metabolism.

Women with mastalgia have been found to have abnormal plasma fatty acid profiles. Treatment with GLA in the form of Efamast, eight capsules (320 mg GLA) daily for 4 months produces a progressive increase towards normal fatty acid profiles. Following a period of treatment, fatty acid profiles fall back to pretreatment levels and this is consistent with observations from clinical studies where mastalgia recurs in up to half of patients who gain a beneficial response to GLA.

Assessment

The first and most important consideration is to exclude any underlying specific cause for the pain. The cyclical nature of the pain and the effects of any treatment are best assessed using pain charts completed each day by the patient. Reassurance has long been recognized as the most important part of the management and, as long ago as 1879, Bilroth wrote that 'friendly advice, reassurance and the banishment and suspicion and fear of dread disease is of great importance'. This involves taking a careful history and performing a full examination of the breast and, if considered appropriate, mammography. If a dominant or discrete lump is present, management is as for any other mass lesion; likewise if there is any suspicious lesion visible on mammography this requires

Table 3.2   Response of drug treatment in cyclical and non-cyclical mastalgia

	% useful response cyclical	non-cyclical	% side-effects
Danazol	79	40	30
GLA	58	38	4
Bromocriptine	54	33	35

appropriate investigation. Thereafter it has been demonstrated that reassurance alone is sufficient for over 85% of patients.

Drugs used in the treatment of mastalgia

Diuretics

There is no scientific rationale for prescribing diuretics for cyclical mastalgia. Double-blind placebo-controlled studies have shown no benefit and these drugs no longer have a place in the management of cyclical breast pain.

Vitamin B6 — pyridoxine

This has been shown to be of some benefit in patients with the premenstrual syndrome. It is possibly of benefit in relief of mild tenderness but in randomized controlled trials has not caused significant improvements, and it is therefore no longer considered an appropriate treatment for breast pain.

Danazol

Danazol is a synthetic steroid with anti-gonadotrophic properties. Its action in humans has not been clearly defined. Although it can inhibit the secretion of luteinizing hormone and follicle stimulating hormone it only does so in the human in very high dosage. It has a local tissue effect and has been shown to bind to both progesterone and androgen receptors but not to oestrogen receptors. Controlled double-blind randomized trials have clearly shown that danazol is beneficial in cyclical mastalgia producing both relief of symptoms and reduction in nodularity at doses as low as 200 mg. It is the most effective agent for severe breast pain and produces improvement in approximately 70% of patients (Table 3.2).

The main problem with danazol is its side-effect profile. There has been a high drop out rate in studies because of these side-effects which include a 5% lowering of voice pitch. This has been permanent in a small number of patients. Other side-effects include hirsuitism and weight gain.

Once a patient's pain is under control with a dose of 200 mg daily then it is usually possible to reduce patients to a maintenance dose of 100 mg daily on alternate days.

GLA

The fatty acid deficiency hypothesis has led to the testing of treatment by supplementing the diet with the EFA GLA. EPO is a natural source of GLA which is prescribed as Efamast. It has proved useful in mild to moderate cyclical mastalgia and, importantly, it has virtually no side-effects. Patient acceptance is high as it is viewed as a natural substance rather than a hormone or a drug. A useful response is obtained in approximately 60% of patients (Table 3.2). The dose is 6–8 capsules per day.

Bromocriptine

This has proved consistently effective in relieving cyclical mastalgia and is as effective as GLA (Table 3.2). Dosage is 2.5 mg twice daily which is introduced slowly increasing the dose over 1–2 weeks. The major problem with bromocriptine is that over 30% of women experience side-effects and in 20% these are severe, the most common being nausea, vomiting and dizziness. These side-effects are reduced by introducing the drug slowly and avoiding a dosage higher than 5 mg/day.

Tamoxifen

At present tamoxifen does not have a product licence for use in breast pain. A small number of studies have assessed its effectiveness in cyclical breast pain and in one small study 71% of patients achieve a reduction in their breast pain when treated with a dose of 20 mg, although side-effects were reported by 26%, the most common complaints being hot flushes and increased vaginal discharge.

Luteinizing hormone releasing hormone (LHRH) analogues

Although this may be effective in over 90% of patients with cyclical mastalgia, unacceptable side-effects follow this treatment and include hot flushes in 87%, headache in 57%, diminished libido in 37%, nausea or vomiting 28% and depression/irritability in 24%. This drug cannot therefore be recommended for routine use in patients with cyclical breast pain. The preparations currently available are also very expensive.

Surgery

A small number of patients who have cyclical breast pain either fail to respond to any treatment or relapse following successive courses of different agents. Some of these patients are improved by bilateral mastectomy and breast reconstruction. Such patients require very careful assessment, often with the help of a psychologist. It is clear that some of those patients who have undergone this operation continue to complain of pain and the current view is that this operation is rarely indicated.

Natural history of cyclical mastalgia

Cyclical pain is often relieved by pregnancy and the menopause. Patients with cyclical pain who start having symptoms at an early age tend to have persistent pain throughout their reproductive life whereas patients who have a late age of onset have a shorter overall duration of pain. Treatment in young patients often, therefore, has to be for prolonged periods. The current aim is to treat young patients with severe mastalgia with short, intermittent bursts rather than continuous periods. Many patients with mastalgia do get spontaneous remission of their symptoms.

Other measures

Some patients appear to benefit from wearing a well-fitting brassiere worn 24 h/day. Between 5% and 15% of patients have pain of such a degree they require specific treatment. Reduction of caffeine intake and a low fat diet have been suggested to be effective in mastalgia, but few studies have scientifically evaluated these measures.

Summary of management of patients with cyclical mastalgia

- Exclude cancer.
- Reassure.
- Define pattern of pain — pain charts.
- Drug treatment
    first line GLA,
    second line danazol,
    third line bromocriptine,
    fourth line tamoxifen and/or LHRH agonists (useful if pain is severe and not responding rapidly to other agents).

NON-CYCLICAL MASTALGIA

Non-cyclical mastalgia is breast pain with a time pattern which is not associated with cyclical ovarian function. It may be continuous but usually has a random time pattern. Non-cyclical mastalgia is associated with a wide range of apparently unrelated events and conditions. These are usually local rather than systemic, that is their cause is located either in the breast or chest wall. Particular benign breast disorders which are strongly associated with non-cyclical mastalgia are periductal mastitis, fat necrosis and sclerosing adenosis. A condition called Tiezte syndrome, where one or more of the costal cartridges posterior to the breast is enlarged, painful and tender, is also a common cause of non-cyclical mastalgia.

Another syndrome which has not been previously well described is that of tenderness in the pectoralis major muscle. The breast can be lifted away from the chest wall without discomfort whereas grasping the edge of the muscle produces severe pain.

Treatment of non-cyclical mastalgia

• Exclude specific causes such as Tietze syndrome and musculoskeletal influences.
• Wear a firm supporting bra 24 h/day.
• Simple analgesia.
• Less than 40% respond to hormonal agents (Table 3.2) — GLA should be the first of these agents tried because of its low incidence of side-effects.

If there is a persistent localized painful area then the use of local anaesthetic and steroid injection is effective in the short term in up to 70%. A useful combination is 40 mg of methylprednisolone combined with 1% lignocaine.

A non-steroidal anti-inflammatory agent may be useful for the group with musculoskeletal pain.

NODULARITY

Nodularity in the breast may be diffuse or focal. As previously noted premenstrual nodularity is such a common finding that it should be considered normal. Generalized nodularity was previously considered to be abnormal and termed fibroadenosis and fibrocystic disease. This is unfortunate since it is now clear that there is little correlation between generalized nodularity and the underlying histological appearances. These terms are, therefore, inappropriate and should no longer be used.

GENERALIZED NODULARITY

Breasts are normally nodular and in almost all instances generalized nodularity is normal.

Management

- Clinical examination.
- Mammography if over 35 years.
- Reassure if no clinical or mammographic abnormality.

In the absence of any clinical or radiological abnormality these patients require reassurance that their breasts are normal and that, as a group, they are no more likely to develop breast cancer than women whose breasts do not have generalized nodularity.

FOCAL NODULARITY

Incidence

This is the most common cause of a breast lump up to the age of 50. Although accounting for up to 70% of breast lumps in women under the age of 40, localized benign nodularity remains a very common cause of a breast lump until after the menopause. Although within an area of localized nodularity there can be areas of localized fibrosis, an increase in the number of glandular elements (adenosis), the presence of small cysts and areas of apocrine change — all these changes are now considered part of normal breast involution; they are also often present in other areas of the same breast which are not nodular and are a common finding in the normal population of women of this age. Localized nodularity is only rarely associated with a focal pathological abnormality such as a localized area of sclerosis, epithelial hyperplasia or a breast cancer.

Management

- Clinical examination.
- Mammography if over 35 years.
- Ultrasound is often of use.
- FNAC if discrete area.
- Biopsy indicated if clinical, cytological or radiological suspicion of malignancy.

Some units biopsy all patients with localized nodularity over the age of 40 who do not have definitive evidence that the lesion is benign — that is those patients who do not have completely lucent mammograms or one or even two FNAC reports which show benign elements only. These women should be reassured and discharged if appropriate investigations show no abnormality. They do not require regular follow up as in some women this increases anxiety.

DISORDERS OF INVOLUTION

Breast involution is usually obvious by the age of 35. The changes include the disappearance of lobular epithelium and specialized lobular connective tissue, with replacement by the more usual fibrous tissue found in the interlobular region. Aberrations of breast involution include macrocyst formation, sclerosis and failure of all breast tissue to involute at the same rate. During involution there can be an increase in the number of cells lining the terminal duct lobular unit — epithelial hyperplasia.

CYSTIC DISEASE OF THE BREAST

Cystic disease of the breast is a term which should be restricted to the clearly defined group of women who present with palpable breast cysts. Terms such as fibrocystic disease and cystic mastopathy should no longer be in clinical use.

Astley Cooper in 1829 first distinguished cysts as separate entities from breast cancer. In the early 1900s workers postulated that cysts arose as a consequence of senile involution of breast lobules and this remains the currently held view of their pathogenesis.

Incidence

Approximately 7% of all women in the western world present at sometime during their life to hospital with a palpable breast cyst. Cysts are most common in the perimenopausal age group and they are uncommon after the menopause (Fig. 2.18, see page 26).

Aetiology of cystic disease

There is considerable indirect evidence that cystic disease is hormonally related — its bilateral nature, its relationship to the menopause and the response of cystic disease to endocrine treatment. There is no convincing direct evidence, however, that women who develop breast cysts have a different profile of plasma hormones to those without cysts. Studies have shown that the levels of EFAs in the plasma of patients with cysts are lower than in the general population.

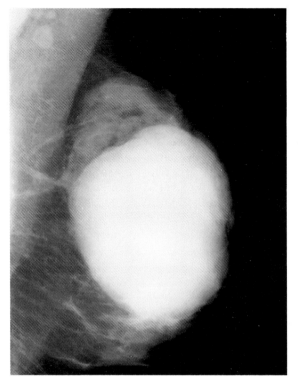

Fig. 3.1 Mammogram of a breast cyst. There is a large mass lesion which is reasonably well localized and in parts is surrounded by a halo.

Clinical aspects of cystic disease

Presentation

The majority of patients present with a smooth discrete breast lump which may be fluctuant. Non-fluctuant, so called 'tension cysts', can clinically resemble a carcinoma. Pain can be a presenting symptom (less than 30%) and cysts can also be discovered incidentally during the screening process (Fig. 3.1). The total number of palpable breast cysts a woman develops varies greatly between individuals; approximately one-half develop only a single cyst, one-third have between two and five cysts and the remainder more than five. Cysts are more common in the left than right breast, as is breast cancer. About one-third of patients have cysts in both breasts.

Management

All patients over 35 years should have a mammogram prior to needle aspiration as 1–3% of patients with cysts have an incidental carcinoma.

- Aspirate with a 21g needle.
- If multiple cysts are present, ultrasound is as specific as aspiration in determining whether the lesions are cystic.
- If fluid is obtained, aspirate cyst to dryness.
- No fluid to cytology unless evenly bloodstained.
- Examine patient after aspiration to determine if residual mass. If mass present requires investigation with cytology, ultrasound and/or biopsy.
- Review patient 3–6 weeks after cyst aspiration to check for refilling. Cysts which rapidly or persistently refill more than twice should be excised as there is an association between repeated and rapid refilling and malignancy.

Risk of carcinoma

Patients who develop palpable breast cysts are at some increased risk (relative risk 1.5–4 times) of developing breast carcinoma. The risk is probably greatest in patients with multiple and bilateral cysts and the order of risk is probably of clinical significance (relative risk approximately 4 times). Debate continues on whether these patients should have earlier and more regular screening than is currently available through the government screening programme.

Treatment of patients with multiple cysts

Some women develop large numbers of cysts with approximately 2% having more than 25 cysts and 1% more than 100 cysts. There is some clinical evidence that danazol reduces cyst formation. In the majority of patients with multiple cysts, no treatment is indicated. In particular these women should not be subjected to regular cyst aspiration as an out-patient. What they require is regular ultrasound and mammographic assessment of their breasts with periodic aspiration of palpable cysts, probably once every 1–2 years. This is most comfortably performed under intravenous sedation.

SCLEROSIS

Sclerosing adenosis, radial scars and complex sclerosing lesions (this term incorporates the lesions previously called sclerosing papillomatosis or duct adenoma and includes infiltrating epitheliosis) are all examples of sclerosis occurring in the period of breast involution. These lesions are important because they cause diagnostic problems to the surgeon, radiologist and pathologist. Sclerosing adenosis and radial scars are both associated with distortion of the terminal duct lobular unit and yet show no significant hyperplasia. Complex sclerosing lesions which are less common are more frequently associated with significant degrees of epithelial hyperplasia.

There is some debate as to whether radial scars might be the precursors of invasive tubular carcinomas although the current view is that these lesions should not be considered premalignant or a significant risk factor for subsequent breast cancer. Areas of sclerosis are best considered aberrations of breast involution and following excision follow up is not required unless the lesion is associated with significant degrees of epithelial hyperplasia.

Clinical features

Patients with these conditions may either present with a breast lump or breast pain, or have an asymptomatic mammographic abnormality detected at a centre which has a screening programme. In such instances they are usually impalpable.

Management

FNAC performed free hand if the lesion is palpable, or stereotactically if impalpable, often indicates that the lesion is benign.

Excisional biopsy is often required to make a definitive diagnosis.

EPITHELIAL HYPERPLASIA

An increase in the number of layers of epithelial cells lining the terminal duct lobular unit is known as epithelial hyperplasia. Previously this change was called epitheliosis or papillomatosis but these terms can now be regarded as obsolete. The degree of hyperplasia can be graded as mild, moderate or florid. Mild hyperplasia which is more than two but not more than four epithelial cells in depth is associated with no greater risk of invasive breast carcinoma than comparable women who do not have this feature.

Clinical significance of epithelial hyperplasia

Patients with moderate and florid degrees of epithelial hyperplasia but which do not have atypical features (proliferative disease without atypia) are considered to have a slightly increased (1.5–2 times) risk of invasive carcinoma relative to comparable women who do not have this feature.

Women who have a lesion which shows a combination of hyperplasia and cellular atypia known as atypical hyperplasia have a risk of developing breast cancer 4–5 times that of the general population and are at moderately increased risk. It is only this order of risk which is considered significant. There is a strong interaction with family history and atypical hyperplasia and it is relevant to consider women with atypical hyperplasia who have a positive family history separately from those who do not. A definition of a positive family history is that at least one first-degree relative – be it mother, daughter, sister – has proven breast cancer.

The clinical significance of epithelial hyperplasia can be best appreciated by the analysis of the proportion of patients with the various lesions who have developed breast cancer during a prolonged follow-up period. This analysis is shown in Figure 3.2 and demonstrates that the absolute risk of breast cancer development in a women with atypical hyperplasia without a family history is 8% at 10 years whereas in those with a positive family history the risk is 20–25% at 15 years. The magnitude of risk for women with atypical hyperplasia and a positive family history is very similar to that for certain types of carcinoma in situ.

Clinical features

Patients with atypical hyperplasia do not present with typical clinical signs which allow a clinical diagnosis to be made and they can present with a lump, lumpiness, nipple discharge, or they can be identified as having either a localized clinical or mammographic abnormality detected by screening. When a fine needle aspirate is performed from an area of moderate or florid hyperplasia with or without atypia, the aspirate is usually markedly cellular and in some instances the cells show atypical features. These lesions are, therefore, usually reported as suspicious or highly suspicious of malignancy on FNAC. Mammographically, areas of hyperplasia may be associated with areas of distortion of architecture, as in a complex sclerosing lesion, or they can be associated with microcalcification and are diagnosed only after a localization biopsy. The majority of epithelial hyperplasias are, however, not associated with any specific symptoms.

Management

- Moderate and florid hyperplasia: no clinically significant risk and therefore no further follow-up required.
- Atypical hyperplasia: determine whether there is a positive family history so the absolute risk can be estimated and discussed with the patient. Options are close clinical and mammographic surveillance or subcutaneous mastectomy with immediate reconstruction.

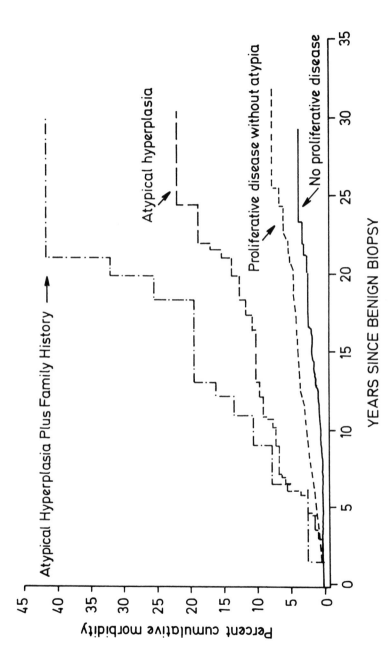

Fig. 3.2   Percentage of patients developing breast cancer after a biopsy showing atypical hyperplasia with or without family history.

RESIDUAL BREAST TISSUE

In some individuals not all breast tissue involutes at the same rate and therefore results in clinical and mammographic asymmetry, and this can sometimes be difficult to differentiate from breast cancer.

Management

FNAC and mammography repeated after an interval of 3–6 months are the best methods of establishing whether an area of clinical nodularity or localized mammographic density are due to this condition.

GYNAECOMASTIA

Growth of breast tissue in males to any extent at all ages is known as gynaecomastia. It is an entirely benign condition and usually reversible. The degree of enlargement varies and in extreme cases the size or shape may be similar to that of the female breast. Histologically the changes are identical to those described in virginal hypertrophy.

Age incidence

Gynaecomastia occurs in three different age groups. The first is found in the neonatal period in which palpable breast tissue transiently develops in 60–90% of all new-born babies because of transplacental passage of oestrogens. Puberty and old age are the other times when gynaecomastia commonly occurs.

Pubertal gynaecomastia

This affects boys between the ages of 10 and 19, with the peak incidence being between the ages of 13 and 14. Some degree of pubertal gynaecomastia occurs in between 30% and 70% of boys if carefully sought. The aetiology and hormonal basis are not completely understood although it is probably due to an oestrogen/androgen imbalance. It usually requires no treatment as 80% spontaneously resolve within 2 years. Occasionally, because it is unsightly and embarrassing subcutaneous mastectomy is indicated. This operation can usually be performed through a small circumareolar incision. During the operation a small disk of breast tissue should be left attached to the undersurface of the areola and some fat should remain on the skin flaps to ensure that the end result is not an unsightly depression in the anterior chest wall.

Table 3.3   Causes of gynaecomastia expressed as a percentage

Cause	%
Puberty	25
Idiopathic (senescent)	25
Drugs (cimetidine, digoxin, spironolactone, androgens or anti-oestrogens)	10–20
Cirrhosis or malnutrition	8
Primary hypogonadism	8
Testicular tumours	3
Secondary hypogonadism	2
Hyperthyroidism	1.5
Renal disease	1

Adult gynaecomastia

Senescent gynaecomastia commonly affects males aged between 50 and 80 years. In the majority it does not appear to be associated with any endocrine abnormality although there may be an underlying luteinizing hormone/follicle stimulating hormone imbalance.

Specific causes of gynaecomastia need to be considered and include drugs, cirrhosis, malnutrition, hypogonadism and testicular tumours. The relative frequency of these different causes is outlined in Table 3.3.

Clinical features of gynaecomastia

Breast lesions are usually soft, involve the whole gland and are commonly bilateral. Unilateral eccentric, tender, hard or ulcerating lesions suggest the underlying pathology may be breast cancer. In these cases mammography is often useful and FNAC will usually indicate if the mass is malignant.

Indications for investigation

Gynaecomastia is common and the finding of non-tender palpable breast tissue on routine examination does not require any evaluation. In most instances a careful history is sufficient to uncover most of the conditions associated with gynaecomastia. If no abnormalities are found on physical examination to explain the gynaecomastia the patient should be re-examined again in 6 months.

A history of recent onset of progressive breast enlargement with or without pain and tenderness without an easily identifiable cause (such as an underlying disease or specific drug therapy) is an indication for investigation. In such instances blood should be taken to assess liver,

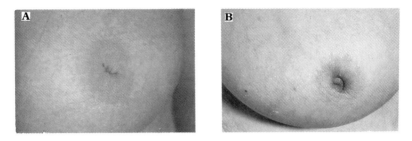

Fig. 3.3 Nipple retraction due to **A** benign (duct ectasia) pathology and to **B** direct involvement with cancer.

renal and thyroid function. If no clear cause is apparent when the results of these investigations are available then blood hormone levels should be measured to exclude a hormone-producing tumour.

NIPPLE ABNORMALITIES

Changes in the nipple can occur with both benign and malignant disease and include: nipple inversion/retraction, nipple discharge and skin changes involving the nipple and areola.

NIPPLE INVERSION/RETRACTION

Nipple inversion is described when the whole nipple is pulled in; and nipple retraction is described when only part of the nipple is pulled in, usually at the site of a single duct to produce a slit-like appearance of the nipple (Fig. 3.3). These changes can be congenital or acquired. The acquired causes in order of frequency are: duct ectasia, carcinoma, periductal mastitis and tuberculosis.

Investigations

All patients with acquired nipple inversion or retraction should have a full clinical examination and if the patient is over the age of 35 a mammogram.

Management

- If no palpable mass or mammograms normal/benign — surgery not indicated unless for cosmetic reasons.
- If mass palpable or mammographic abnormality evident — FNAC or biopsy and duct excision indicated.

NIPPLE DISCHARGE

The causes of nipple discharge in order of frequency are: physiological, duct papilloma, duct ectasia, periductal mastitis, cancer and galactorrhoea. Nipple discharge can be from single or multiple ducts. Single duct discharge is more likely to be serious than multiple duct discharge. Physiological discharge is very common and can be obtained by massage of the breasts in up to two-thirds of patients. The amount of discharge is variable and is, characteristically, intermittent from multiple ducts and usually requires massage to produce it.

Milky discharge from a single duct is common and usually physiological. Galactorrrhoea occurs from multiple ducts in both breasts and is usually associated with a raised plasma prolactin level. Bromocriptine is effective in stopping this milk flow but should be used after exclusion of a pituitary tumour (galactorrhoea and a prolactin greater than five times the upper limit of normal need investigation).

A plan for the investigation of nipple discharge is shown in figure 2.14.

CHANGES IN SKIN OF NIPPLE AND AREOLA

These can be due to eczema, Paget's disease or can occur as a direct result by infiltration of an underlying carcinoma. Patients should have the same investigations as for nipple inversion/retraction.

Management

- Where there is a mass lesion or mammographic abnormality detected this should be appropriately investigated.
- If there is no mass lesion but Paget's disease is considered a possible diagnosis then a portion of the nipple or areolar skin should be excised under local anaesthetic and submitted for histological examination.
- Eversion of the nipple can often be satisfactorily performed under local anaesthesia by incising the ducts and loosely placing two horizontal mattress sutures of chromic catgut to maintain eversion whilst healing occurs. If the nipple inversion is marked and longstanding, a total duct excision is required to evert the nipple.

FAT NECROSIS

Fat necrosis of the breast was first described as a clinical entity in 1920. It accounts for approximately one in 200 of all breast problems.

Aetiology and pathogenesis

Fat necrosis was originally thought to be secondary to trauma and it is often called 'traumatic fat necrosis'. In fact a history of trauma is present in less that 40% of patients. Nowadays it is often seen after road traffic accidents as a result of seat belt trauma of the breast.

Clinical features

Fat necrosis is of clinical concern because it is sometimes difficult to distinguish from carcinoma on both physical examination and mammography. Characteristically there is a painless mass in the breast which is firm, ill defined and poorly mobile. Associated skin thickening or retraction are often seen and this increases the clinical suspicion that the lesion may be malignant. It can occur anywhere in the breast but it is most common in the subareolar region. Following resolution fat cysts may remain in the breast.

Management

- If there is a definite history of trauma and overlying bruising and a palpable mass is present, then management should be initially by observation.
- It is important to note there may be an initial increase in size of the mass.
- FNAC and mammography should be performed.
- If suspicion of malignancy persists a biopsy is indicated.

BREAST HAEMATOMA

Haematoma is the most common breast problem following trauma. This may be major trauma following a road traffic accident or local trauma from an aspirate or fine needle aspirate, core needle or open biopsy. The mammographic appearance of a haematoma may be ominous with poorly defined margins raising the possibility of a carcinoma. Because it is known that haematomas can follow FNAC, and that these may mimic cancer, it is now practice to perform mammography prior to FNAC.

In extremely unusual circumstances breast carcinoma may present with spontaneous haemorrhage and a haematoma in the absence of breast trauma. Ultrasound can be useful in the diagnosis of a breast haematoma.

Breast haematoma may also occur spontaneously in patients on anticoagulant therapy.

Management

- Small haematomas following direct trauma or needle aspiration are treated with support, analgesia and observation.
- Large haematomas occurring spontaneously with evidence of overlying skin thinning or following surgery may need formal drainage.

It is important to appreciate that some patients with breast cancer present with a recent history of trauma. Failure of a haematoma to resolve rapidly, particularly after a fine needle aspirate which has failed to provide diagnostic information is an indication for open biopsy.

GALACTOCELE

This is a cystic lesion occurring in women during or after pregnancy or breast feeding. It contains breast milk which may be inspissated. It is said to be more frequent in women who stop breast feeding suddenly. Treatment is by aspiration which both confirms the diagnosis and usually cures the condition.

BLOCKED MONTGOMERY'S TUBERCULES

These glands on the surface of the areola can become obstructed and the sebaceous secretion builds up and presents as a periareolar lump which if troublesome can be excised.

BENIGN NEOPLASMS

Duct papilloma

These lesions can be single or multiple. They are very common and because of their frequency it has been suggested that they might best be considered as aberrations rather than true benign neoplasms. They show minimal if any malignant potential. There is some debate whether patients with the so-called 'multiple papilloma syndrome' are at increased risk of subsequent breast cancer although this is disputed.

Symptoms

The most frequent symptom is spontaneous nipple discharge which can be serous or bloodstained. Even serous discharges from patients with a duct papilloma are usually positive for blood on 'stix testing. Occasionally in large papillomas the patients also present with a breast mass.

Clinical features

Characteristically the discharge emanates from a single duct. As there is often duct dilatation distal to the papilloma, pressure over the dilated duct at the areola margin produces large amounts of discharge. The discharge itself is usually either bloodstained or is positive for blood on testing. Occasionally a palpable mass is present at the areola margin which can represent either the papilloma itself or the dilated duct beyond.

Management

- Perform mammography.
- Test for blood.
- If positive for blood or the discharge is persistent or troublesome the patient may require excision of the involved duct.

Treatment

Excision of a duct or 'microdochectomy' can be performed through a very small circumareolar incision. As the majority of causes of duct discharge occur within the first 2 cm of the major subareolar duct it is usually only necessary to excise a small portion of the diseased duct.

LIPOMAS

Lipomas are common both within the subcutaneous tissue over the breast and within the breast. The main interest in this lesion lies in the confusion with a 'pseudolipoma' which is a soft mass which can be felt around a small breast cancer caused by indrawing of the fat by a spiculated carcinoma.

Clinical presentation

Patients present with a soft lobulated, localized mass in the subcutaneous tissue or within the breast itself.

Management

- Establish diagnosis by mammography/FNAC.
- Excise only if suspicion of malignancy or if troublesome.

COSMETIC SURGERY

Breast augmentation

Indications

Although these include breast asymmetry resulting from congenital anomalies, the main reason for patients requesting breast augmentation is a desire to increase the size of their breasts. There are few operations in which it is more difficult to evaluate the outcome. The operation itself produces a remarkable degree of happiness and there is almost uniform improvement in self image. Only 1% of women who have had this operation performed say that they are unhappy with the result and would not have it performed again.

Technique

Most patients can be adequately treated by insertion of a prosthesis placed either under the breast tissue itself or under the pectoralis major muscle. For patients who have small truncated breasts which lack tissue in all dimensions (known as tuberous or tubular breasts), it is often necessary to insert a tissue expander initially and then replace this with a permanent prosthesis.

Prostheses and their problems

A variety of materials have been used to increase the size of the breast. These include silicone implants, saline-filled prostheses and a combination of both. Saline-filled prostheses are associated with a high rate of saline leakage (more than 15%) with subsequent spontaneous deflation and this has thrown these into disfavour. Double lumen prostheses are difficult to fabricate and have many potential problems. Currently the best cosmetic results are obtained with a silicone gel-filled prosthesis. There is no evidence, clinical or otherwise, of carcinogenesis resulting from their use. At present there is no conclusive proof that they cause autoimmune disease, but the increasing number of anecdotal reports of connective tissue disease in women who have been the recipients of such implants merits further investigation. A prospective registration programme for patients undergoing augmentation has been introduced to try and resolve this problem.

Postoperative technical and mechanical problems such as implant deflation, perforation, rupture, creasing or palpable folds may occasionally be encountered. Other complications of such surgery include capsular contracture and, rarely, infection. These complications may require surgical revision and removal or exchange of the implant but do not in themselves make breast implants dangerous. The consensus view is that silicone breast implants are safe.

The most common postoperative complication of augmentation and reconstructive mammoplasty using silicone prostheses is the formation of, and subsequent contraction of, fibrous capsules around implants. Capsule formation around an implant is universal and has been reported with all types, shapes, surfaces and sizes of prostheses. The reported incidence of clinically significant capsular contracture ranges from 3–74%, this variation reflecting different methods of measurement. It appears to occur less commonly with saline-filled implants than with gel-filled ones. There is some evidence that textured implants which have an irregular surface reduce contracture rates; in one study they decreased the incidence of capsular contracture at 1 year from 58% to 8%. The majority of implants used in the UK at the present time are, therefore, textured silicone gel-filled prostheses.

Much publicity has surrounded the 'bleed' of silicone gel from the prosthesis. It has been known for some time that minute amounts of silicone gel leak or bleed through the envelope of prostheses and can migrate to other organs. There is no evidence that the silicone gel bleed is either responsible for the capsule formation or causes problems when it migrates to other organs.

Reduction mammoplasty

Indications

The reasons for performing reduction mammoplasty include juvenile hypertrophy, generally large breasts and to achieve symmetry in patients with asymmetrical breasts resulting from either congenital anomalies or surgery. One common indication for reduction mammoplasty is to reduce the size of one breast to match the size of a contralateral reconstructed breast following mastectomy for breast cancer. Patients need to be informed of the scars that will result from this surgery and possible complications.

The complications that follow this type of surgery relate to wound healing, scarring, infection and haematoma formation.

Technique

Breast reduction is accomplished by maintaining the nipple and areola on a pedicle of breast tissue and re-siting it after excision of skin and breast tissue. The new site for the nipple/areola complex is carefully marked prior to operation (Fig. 3.4), the skin is then mobilized from the underlying breast tissue and the bulk of breast reduced

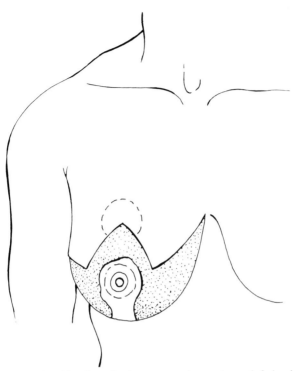

Fig. 3.4 Lines of incision for reduction mammoplasty using an inferior dermal flap technique; the dotted line superiorly represents the new position of the nipple.

circumferentially around the nipple/areola pedicle. Scars resulting from this procedure leave an inverted T pattern.

Mastopexy ('breast lift')

Ptosis (sagging) of the breast is common following pregnancy. Mastopexy is indicated where there is severe ptosis and is commonly called 'a breast lift'.

Technique

Simple nipple/areola advancement will help but usually some skin excision either by removal of a V-shaped portion of skin inferiorly, or an excision of skin as in reduction mammoplasty are required. A mastopexy can be combined with an augmentation to fill out the loose skin and replace some of the breast tissue which has disappeared.

4. Breast infection

INTRODUCTION

Breast infection is much less common than it used to be. It is seen occasionally in neonates but most commonly affects adult females between the ages of 18 and 50. In the adult breast infection can be considered as lactational or non-lactational. Infection can also affect the skin overlying the breast and can occur either as a primary event or secondary to a lesion within the skin such as a sebaceous cyst or to an underlying condition such as hidradenitis suppurativa. The organisms responsible for different types of breast infection and the most appropriate antibiotics for treating these organisms are summarized in Table 4.1. The guiding principles in treating breast infection are:

• Antibiotics should be given early to abort abscess formation.
• Hospital referral is indicated if the infection does not settle rapidly with antibiotics.
• If an abscess is suspected this should be confirmed by aspiration.

Table 4.1 Organisms responsible for different types of breast infection and appropriate antibiotics

Type of infection	Organism	Antibiotic No penicillin allergy	Penicillin allergy
Neonatal Lactating Skin associated	*Staph. aureus*	Flucloxacillin	Erythromycin
Non-lactating	*Staph. aureus* Enterococci Anaerobic streptococci *Bacteroides species*	Augmentin	Combination of cephradine or erythromycin and metronidazole

● If the lesion is solid on aspiration then a sample of cells should be obtained for cytology to exclude an underlying inflammatory carcinoma (Fig. 4.1).

Specific infections affecting the breast can be defined.

MASTITIS NEONATORUM

Aetiology and pathogenesis

Continued enlargement of the breast bud in the first week or two of life occurs in about 60% of new-born babies and the gland may reach several centimetres in size before regressing. Although *Staphylococcus aureus* (*Staph. aureus*) is the usual organism, *Escherichia coli* can sometimes cause this infection.

Clinical features

Neonatal breast buds are usually red and somewhat tender but infection is uncommon. When infection is present the breast bud becomes hard, tender and erythematous. Abscess formation can follow and some infants become severely ill.

Management

If an abscess develops, incision and drainage should be performed under general anaesthetic and combined with intravenous antibiotics. The incision should be made as peripherally as possible.

LACTATING BREAST INFECTION

Puerperal mastitis and lactating breast abscesses are now uncommon in developed countries but are still frequent problems in many parts of the world. The reasons for the decrease in frequency are improved maternal and infant hygiene, changes in breast feeding patterns and earlier treatment of infection with appropriate antibiotics. *Staph. aureus* is usually the organism responsible although *Staph. epidermis* and streptococci are occasionally isolated.

Aetiology and pathogenesis

It remains uncertain whether the organisms responsible for lactating breast infection are derived from the skin of the patient herself or from the mouth of her suckling child. Infection is usually associated with a break in the skin, such as a cracked nipple. These skin breaks reduce local defence mechanisms and result in an increase in the number of bacteria in the area around the nipple. These bacteria then enter the breast through the nipple and not through breaks in the skin as has been previously suggested. When infection is present the involved portion of breast is often engorged with milk and drainage into major ducts is then poor. Whether problems with milk drainage result from blockage of a major breast duct or occur as a consequence of infection is unknown.

Clinical features

Infection associated with breast feeding is most common within the first month after delivery, although some women do develop infection associated with weaning. Presenting features include pain, swelling and tenderness (Fig. 4.2). In the later stages there may be a fluctuant mass with overlying shiny, red skin. Axillary lymphadenopathy is not usually a feature of lactating breast infection. Patients can be toxic with a pyrexia, tachycardia and leucocytosis.

Management

- Antibiotics administered early in puerperal mastitis can abort abscess formation. Tetracycline, ciprofloxacin and chloramphenicol should not be used as they enter breast milk and may do the child harm. Breast feeding should be continued as this promotes drainage of the engorged segment and helps resolve infection.
- As fluctuation can be a late sign of abscess formation, patients whose condition does not rapidly improve on antibiotic therapy should have needle aspiration performed over the point of maximum tenderness following application of a local anaesthetic (EMLA) cream which is left in situ for 1 h. There are two main options available for the management of women with lactating breast infection whether it is clinically evident or diagnosed on aspiration.

Treatment plan for lactating abscesses

Apply local anaesthetic (EMLA) 2–4 g leave in situ for 1 h

?state of skin overlying abscess

Normal → Thinned or necrotic

Aspirate with 19g needle
Continue oral antibiotics

Incision with 15 blade
irrigate with normal saline

Repeat aspiration, two or three per week, until no further pus aspirated

Daily irrigation until resolution

Few lactating abscesses require drainage under general anaesthesia and the placement of a drain after incision and drainage is not necessary. Patients who have incision and drainage of their breast abscess under general anaesthesia usually have to stop breast feeding, but patients who are treated by mini-incision or aspiration and antibiotics can continue to breast feed if they wish. It is rarely necessary to suppress lactation in patients with breast infection.

NON-LACTATING INFECTION

These infections can be separated into those occurring centrally in the periareolar region and those affecting the peripheral breast tissue.

Periareolar infection

This predominantly affects young women with a mean age of 32 years. Histologically it is characterized by active inflammation around non-dilated ducts. The predominant cell in the periductal inflammation is usually the plasma cell, which explains why plasma cell mastitis is one of the terms which has been used for this condition. It is unfortunate that the most common term in clinical use for this condition is duct ectasia as patients who have active periductal inflammation have little evidence of ectatic or dilated ducts. Duct ectasia appears to be a separate clinical and pathological entity which affects an older age group and is characterized by duct dilatation with minimal periductal inflammation.

Aetiology and pathogenesis

Current evidence suggests that smoking is an important factor in the aetiology of this condition. How smoking results in damage to the subareolar breast ducts is unknown. Bacteria including enterococci, anaerobic streptococci, *Bacteroides species* and *Staph. aureus* have been isolated from the lesions of periductal mastitis and also play some role in its aetiology and pathogenesis.

Clinical features

Patients may present initially with periareolar inflammation with or without a mass (Fig. 4.3) or an established abscess (Fig. 4.4). Associated features include central breast pain, nipple retraction at the site of the diseased duct and nipple discharge. Periareolar inflammatory masses associated with periductal mastitis account for 3–4% of all benign breast masses.

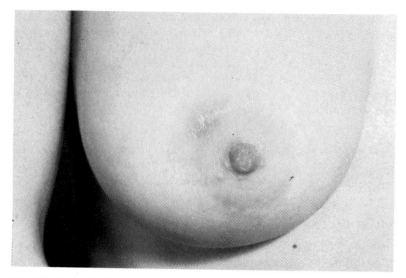

Fig. 4.3 Periareolar inflammation secondary to periductal mastitis.

Management

- Initial treatment is with appropriate antibiotics.
- If the mass fails to resolve, perform fine needle aspirate to exclude an underlying cancer and an ultrasound to determine if an abscess is present.
- If an abscess is present, treat as for a lactating abscess.

Infection associated with periductal mastitis is frequently recurrent because treatment by incision and drainage or aspiration does not remove the underlying diseased duct. In up to one-third of patients a mammary duct fistula follows incision and drainage of a periareolar breast abscess.

Treatment for recurrent episodes of periareolar sepsis is excision of the diseased duct by an experienced breast surgeon, the operation being performed under antibiotic cover.

MAMMARY DUCT FISTULA

Mammary duct fistula is a communication between the skin usually in the periareolar region and a major subareolar breast duct (Fig. 4.5).

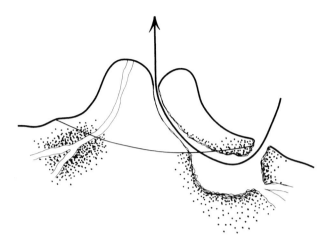

Fig. 4.5 A schematic diagram of a mammary duct fistula. At one side of the diagram a duct can be seen surrounded by numbers of black dots which represent periareolar inflammation. A biopsy of this area, incision and drainage if an abscess develops or spontaneous discharge usually at the areolar margin results in a mammary duct fistula seen on the other side of the diagram. Note the retracted nipple at the site of the involved duct.

Aetiology and pathogenesis

Periductal mastitis is the major cause of mammary duct fistula and may develop following: incision and drainage of a non-lactating breast abscess; spontaneous discharge of a periareolar inflammatory mass; biopsy of an area of periductal mastitis; or incision and drainage of a non-lactating breast abscess.

Clinical features

There is a discharging fistula at the areolar margin usually associated with nipple retraction. The median age of patients with this problem is 35 years and over 90% are smokers. There have usually been preceding episodes of recurrent abscess formation and pussy discharge both through the nipple and through the fistula opening at the areolar margin. Occasionally there can be more than one opening at the areolar margin from a single involved duct.

Management

Treatment is surgical and consists of either opening up the fistula tract and leaving it to granulate, or excising the fistula and closing the wound primarily under antibiotic cover.

PERIPHERAL NON-LACTATING BREAST ABSCESSES

Aetiology and pathogenesis

Peripheral non-lactating breast abscesses are less common than peri-areolar abscesses, but they do occur and are often associated with an underlying disease state such as diabetes, rheumatoid arthritis, steroid treatment and trauma; they can also be associated with sebaceous cysts within the skin of the breast. Pilonidal abscesses in sheep shearers and barbers have also been reported. *Staph. aureus* is the usual causative organism but some abscesses contain anaeorbic organisms.

Clinical features

These abscesses are more common in premenopausal than postmenopausal women with a ratio of 3:1. Characteristically the patient presents with a lump which is tender and may be associated with inflammatory changes in the overlying skin of the breast. Systemic evidence of malaise or fever are usually absent. There may be a history of an underlying disease process and, if the abscess is secondary to a sebaceous cyst, a punctum may be identified.

Management

As for lactating periareolar abscesses with aspiration (Fig. 4.6) or incision and drainage.

SKIN ASSOCIATED INFECTIONS

Cellulitis of the skin of the breast with or without abscess formation is common, particularly in obese patients and/or those with large breasts. It also affects those who have poor breast hygiene. The lower half of the breast is most commonly affected, where the patient sweats and intertrigo develops. *Staph. aureus* and fungi are the most common organisms responsible for this infection. Skin infection can also be seen in association with sebaceous cysts and hidradenitis suppurativa.

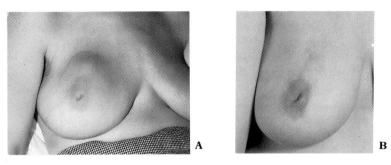

Fig. 4.6 Peripheral breast abscess before (**A**) and after (**B**) treatment by recurrent aspiration and oral antibiotics.

Treatment

- Weight reduction.
- Keep areas as clean and dry as possible — washing twice per day; avoid creams and talcum powder; use cotton bras or cotton T-shirt, or vest worn inside bra.
- Appropriate courses of antibiotics and antifungal powder.

OTHER RARE INFECTIONS

Tuberculosis

Tuberculosis is now rare and can be primary or secondary, but the latter is more common. In secondary tuberculosis infection usually reaches the breast by lymphatic spread from axillary, mediastinal or cervical nodes, or from directly underlying structures such as rib and costochondral junction or pleura.

Clinical features

Tuberculosis predominantly affects women in the latter part of the childbearing period. As it is now rare in developed countries the diagnosis is difficult to make. A breast or axillary sinus is present in up to 50% of patients. The most common presentation is with an acute abscess which occurs as a result of infection of an area of tuberculosis by pyogenic organisms.

Management

- Establish diagnosis — may need biopsy.
- Combination of surgery and antituberculous drug therapy.

Syphilis, actinomycosis, mycotic, helminthic and viral infections occasionally affect the breast, but are rare.

Granulomatous lobular mastitis

This is probably a variant of periductal mastitis and is characterized by non-caseating granulomata and microabscesses confined to the breast.

Clinical features

Young parous women are most frequently affected. Organisms may be found in these lesions but do not appear to have a primary role in its aetiology.

Management

The diagnosis can often be established on fine needle aspiration cytology (FNAC) and surgery should be avoided if possible. When surgical intervention is performed it is frequently followed by wound infection and, occasionally, a mammary duct fistula develops. There is a strong tendency for this condition to persist and recur. There is no specific treatment and the condition usually resolves spontaneously. The same antibiotics used in periductal mastitis have been tried without much success and corticosteroids have been advocated by some.

Factitial disease

Factitious abscesses may be seen in a few patients. These patients generally have psychiatric problems, but some can be quite plausible and the condition needs to be suspected where peripheral abscesses persist or recur after appropriate treatment.

DUCT ECTASIA

Definition and terminology

The conditions of periductal mastitis and duct ectasia, which are benign conditions affecting major breast ducts, are poorly understood and, unfortunately, the terms are often used interchangeably. It is now appreciated that there are almost certainly two separate conditions: periductal mastitis which affects predominantly young women; and duct ectasia which is probably an aberration of normal breast involution which affects older women. It is the same condition that was first recognized in 1923 by Bloodgood when he referred to the variceal tumour of the breast because of the finding of palpable subareolar dilated ducts.

Incidence

Mammary duct ectasia is more common than is generally appreciated and in one autopsy series was found in 25% of normal female breasts. In the majority it does not produce any specific symptoms.

Clinical presentation

Patients can present with nipple discharge, nipple retraction, or a palpable mass which may be hard or doughy. Nipple discharge, often from several ducts, is common and may be profuse and variable in colour. It is the most common cause of nipple discharge in women over the age of 55 years. The discharge is often described as cheesy, being thick and white. Nipple retraction may be the sole presenting feature or be present in association with nipple discharge. Nipple retraction is classically slit like (Fig. 3.3a) and a portion of the nipple is pulled in rather than the whole nipple. This separates it from nipple inversion which is seen either in association with severe inflammatory disease or malignancy (Fig. 3.3b). The mean age of patients with this symptom is 53 years and the retraction is bilateral in 15%. 3–4% of all benign breast masses are related to duct ectasia.

Pathology

The major subareolar ducts are dilated, contain inspissated material and have minimal surrounding inflammation. This contrasts with the picture of periductal mastitis where duct dilatation is absent and periductal inflammation prominent.

Management

Patients whose discharge is troublesome or in whom there is clinical and/or mammographic suspicion of malignancy require surgical excision. Surgery is also indicated in a patient with nipple retraction if there is an associated mass or mammographic abnormality. Otherwise no specific treatment is needed. Patients with duct ectasia presenting with a breast mass are managed in a similar way to any other patient presenting with a breast mass — being investigated by mammography, cytology and, if appropriate, excision.

Operations for duct ectasia

Some patients with duct ectasia will have a single duct discharge and if this is bloodstained they will require excision of the discharging duct to establish the cause. In the majority of patients with duct ectasia, however, it is evident at the time of operation that a number of subareaolar ducts are dilated. In such patients the most appropriate treatment is total duct excision. In this operation all the ducts are divided from behind the nipple and a 1 cm portion of central ducts excised. This is termed a Hadfield's operation in the UK and goes under a variety of synonyms abroad.

Complications

Complications from surgery are rare. Loss of nipple sensation has been reported after total duct excision, but the incidence of this complication can be reduced by performing a total duct excision through a small incision which divides few nerves. Infective complications are infrequent, in contrast to surgery for periductal mastitis.

Breast cancer

5. Risk factors, screening and prevention

INTRODUCTION

Breast cancer is common, affecting one in 12 women and causing 21 000 deaths a year in the UK. The prevalence is around five times higher, and more than 70% of those with 'operable' disease will be alive and well 5 years after diagnosis.

The Government has highlighted breast cancer as one of four 'key sites' in the cancer section of the recent plan of Health for the Nation. They intend to reduce the incidence of breast cancer detected through screening by 25% before the year 2000 (from 98 cases detected per 10 000 screened to 74). They are encouraging those responsible for health care provision to extend the models of care developed for the screened population to the general, symptomatic patient.

Breast cancer is an emotive subject and there is a general fear that all lumps are malignant. This is not so — only one in eight breast lumps presenting to breast clinics are cancers.

Breast diseases, including cancer, are increasingly being treated in specialist units where close co-operation between interested surgeons, pathologists, radiologists and associated staff allow rapid and accurate diagnosis with appropriate treatment to be offered to patients. The trend for breast reconstruction and chemotherapy to be provided in the District General Hospital setting is also increasing with the patient needing to travel only for radiotherapy services. There are plans for specialist training for those interested in breast surgery and there is a move to appoint a specialist breast nurse (counsellor) to every health authority.

HISTORY

Breast cancer is not a new disease and was recorded by the Egyptians. Hippocrates and Celsus both describe some of the clinical features. Leonides was operating on malignant breast lumps at the end of the

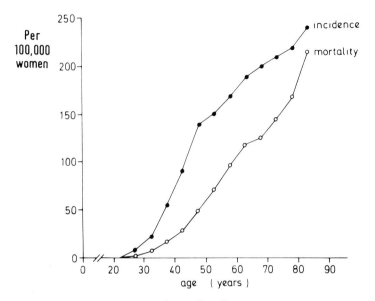

Fig. 5.1   Age-specific incidence and mortality of breast cancer.

first century AD using cautery to both control bleeding and to eradicate remnants of the disease. Galen (c. 130AD) exerted much influence on medical thought and laid down criteria for operative and conservative management; his ideas held sway until the 16th century.

The patron saint of breast diseases is St Agatha, who was martyred having her breasts removed in Sicily, in the third century. There is an extensive literature relating to breast cancer in the Middle Ages and the Renaissance with details of both conventional and some quite bizarre treatments (see Further reading).

RISK FACTORS FOR AND EPIDEMIOLOGY OF BREAST CANCER

Age

The risk of developing breast cancer increases with age. It is rare before the age of 25 but the incidence increases leading up to the menopause, following which there is a slight downward trend during the menopausal years (the menopausal hook of Clemmenson) before its incidence again continues to rise with advancing years although with a reduced rate (Fig. 5.1). Breast cancer accounts for almost 20% of all cancer deaths but, because of variations in the age distribution of different cancers,

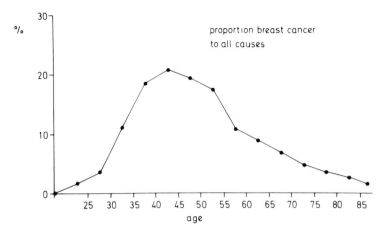

Fig. 5.2 Percentage of all deaths at different ages due to breast cancer.

the proportion of deaths in different ages caused by breast cancer is highest between the ages of 44 and 50 following which it steadily declines (Fig. 5.2).

Geographic variation

There is a marked variation in the incidence of mortality of breast cancer between different countries (Fig. 5.3). Large increases in the rates of breast cancer occur in populations migrating from nations with a low incidence to those with a high incidence of breast cancer, indicating the existence of environmental factors.

Age at menarche and menopause

Women who start menstruating early in life or who have late menopause have an increased risk of developing breast cancer. Women who have a natural menopause after the age of 55 years have twice the risk of developing breast cancer when compared to women whose menopause occurs before the age of 45. In the extreme, women who undergo a bilateral oophorectomy before the age of 35 have 40% the risk of breast cancer of women who have a natural menopause (Table 5.1).

Age at first pregnancy

Nulliparity and late age at first birth both increase the lifetime incidence of breast cancer. The risk of breast cancer in women who have their

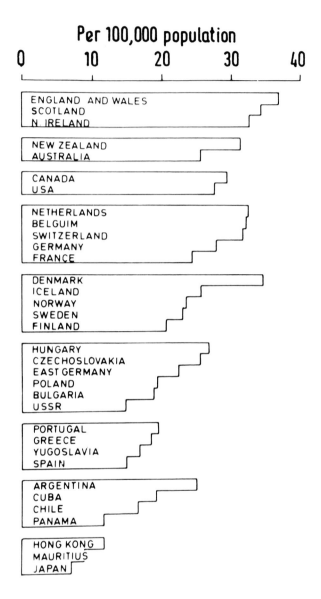

Fig. 5.3   Female breast cancer mortality incidence in different parts of the world.

Table 5.1 Established and probable risk factors for breast cancer

Risk factor	Comparison category	Risk category	Typical relative risk
Age at menarche	16 years	11–14 years	1.3
		15 years	1.1
Age at menopause	45–54 years	After 55 years	1.5
		Before 45 years	0.7
		Oophorectomy before 35 years	0.4
Age at birth of first child	Before 20 years	20–24 years	1.3
		25–29 years	1.6
		30 years	1.9
		Nulliparous	1.9
Family history of breast cancer	No first-degree relatives affected	Mother affected before age of 60	2.0
		Mother affected after age of 60	1.4
		Two first-degree relatives affected	4.0–6.0
Benign breast disease	No evidence of proliferative change	Proliferation only	2.0
		Atypical hyper-plasia	4.5
Alcohol use	Non-drinker	1 drink/day	1.4
		2 drinks/day	1.7
		3 drinks/day	2.0
Radiation	No special exposure	Atomic bomb (100 rad)	3.0
		Repeated fluoro-scopy	1.5–2.0
Oral contraceptive use	Never used	Current use*	1.5
		Prolonged use before first pregnancy	2.0
		Past use*	1.0
Postmenopausal oestrogen replace-ment therapy	Never used	Current use all ages	1.4
		Age < 55 years	1.2
		Age 50–59 years	1.5
		Age 60 years	2.1
		Past use	1.0

* Relative risks may be higher for women with a diagnosis of breast cancer before the age of 40

first child after the age of 30 is about twice that of women who have their first child before the age of 20; women who have their first child after the age of 35 appearing to be at even higher risk than nulliparous women (Table 5.1). An earlier age at the birth of a second child further reduces the risk of breast cancer.

Lactation

Current studies suggest that lactation does reduce breast cancer incidence — breast feeding for at least 3 months reducing the risks of breast cancer by 22% per baby fed.

Family history

When compared with the risk among women having no first-degree relatives with breast cancer, women with a first-degree relative have an elevated risk of the order of 1.5–2 times. This risk may be from 4–6 times higher for those with two affected first-degree relatives, and the risks are heightened if the breast cancer in the affected relative is bilateral. For women who have a sister with bilateral breast cancer which developed before the age of 50, the lifetime cumulative risk appears to be greater than 50% and is even higher if the sister was affected before the age of 40. For women whose mother has unilateral breast cancer after the age of 60, the excess relative risk is only about 40% greater than that associated with having no first-degree relatives with breast cancer.

In certain families it is clear that breast cancer is hereditary, and in 40% of these families there is a mutation in a gene on chromosome 17, the gene being known as the BRCa1. When the gene is cloned it will be possible to offer genetic screening for women with a family history of breast cancer.

Previous benign breast disease

Breast lobules start to involute after the age of 30 and involution is usually well advanced by the menopause although active lobules are often seen in breasts, even in postmenopausal women. The earliest sign of an increase in epithelial activity within the lobular unit is hyperplasia — the epithelial cells lining the terminal ductules enlarging and becoming more numerous. This change does not necessarily progress; but in some women epithelial hyperplasia becomes excessive and the cells develop abnormal features with an irregular pattern of growth. This stage is known as atypical hyperplasia. Although this change only rarely develops into malignancy it would appear that it is a step in that direction. Women with palpable breast cysts, duct papillomas, sclerosing adenosis and moderate/florid epithelial hyperplasia do have some slight increase in the risk of breast cancer compared with those without these changes, but this risk is not of the order that is clinically significant. Patients with hyperplasia and cellular atypia (atypical hyperplasia) do have an increased risk of approximately four to five times (Tables 5.1

Table 5.2   Relative risk for invasive breast cancer in patients with benign disease

Risk	Disease type
No increased risk	Mild hyperplasia
	Duct ectasia
	Apocrine metaplasia
	Fibroadenoma
	Microcysts
	Periductal mastitis
	Adenosis
Slight increased risk	Gross cysts
1.5–2 times	Moderate and florid hyperplasia
	Papilloma
	Sclerosing adenosis
Moderately increased risk	Atypical hyperplasia
4–5 times	

and 5.2). The combination of family history and atypical change is discussed in chapter 3.

Weight

Obesity is not an important risk factor for breast cancer and among premenopausal women it is actually associated with reduced incidence.

Diet

Evidence implicating diet in the aetiology of breast cancer includes the observation that fat may cause mammary tumours in rodents, and that mortality from breast cancer in different countries strongly correlates with the corresponding per capita fat consumption. Studies of total fat have, however, not found that women with breast cancer report a significantly higher consumption than controls, and the relationship may simply reflect total calorific intake rather than just fat intake. No definitive conclusion can therefore be drawn from the data currently available. Some studies have suggested that green vegetables may have a protective effect against breast cancer but this requires confirmation.

Alcohol intake

Alcohol consumption, even at the level of one drink per day, has been associated with a moderate increased risk of breast cancer in the majority of studies (Table 5.1).

Radiation

Exposure to ionizing radiation, particularly between puberty and the age of 30, can substantially increase the risk of breast cancer. However, exposure to clinically important levels is rare.

Oral contraceptive pill

There is no consistent correlation between oral contraceptives and breast cancer risk when one compares the populations who have ever used and never used the pill. In studies of long-term use in young women the majority have shown some elevation of risk; this order of risk appears to be related to the duration of contraceptive pill use before the first full-term pregnancy — the relative risk for long-term use varying between 1.2 and 4.9, with an average of 2 times. This excess risk appears to be limited to women below the ages of 40.

Postmenopausal oestrogen replacement therapy

Use of hormone replacement therapy (HRT) appears to increase the risk of breast cancer by about 40%, and this risk disappears after stopping these preparations. This relative risk (1.4) of developing breast cancer is offset by the benefits of prophylaxis against osteoporosis and ischaemic heart disease. Current cost-benefit analysis indicates that up to 10 years HRT has significant advantages. Data on more prolonged use are scanty but do suggest that there may be a significant risk of breast cancer in women who are on hormone replacement beyond 15 years. Combining progesterone with oestrogen replacement reduces the risk of endometrial cancer but does not appear to decrease the risk of breast cancer and may even add to it.

HRT should probably be used with caution in women who have a relative risk of greater than two for whatever reason (Table 5.1). This recommendation has to be tempered if the symptoms being experienced are such that the quality of a woman's life is miserable. HRT may then be justified after discussion of the risk with the patient. It should not be used as first-line therapy in these women and other measures such as clonidine, Efamast, herbal and homeopathic remedies should be tried first. Progestogens alone may provide some benefit and do not have the same risk as oestrogen alone.

Cigarette smoking

Current evidence suggests there may be a small negative link between breast cancer incidence and smoking but any effect is very small.

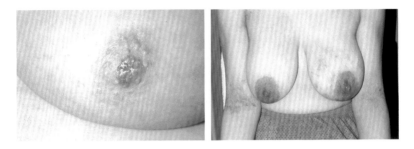

Fig. 2.3 A Paget's disease of the nipple; **B** eczema of the nipple.

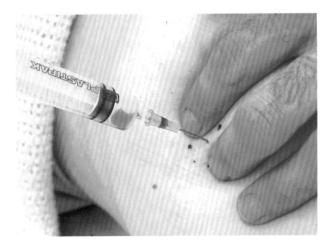

Fig. 2.11 The technique of fine needle aspiration cytology.

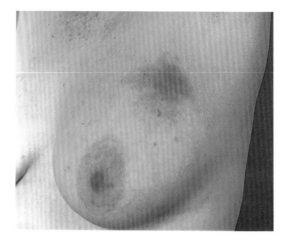

Fig. 4.1 An inflammatory carcinoma of the left breast. The diagnosis was established by FNAC which has caused some bruising.

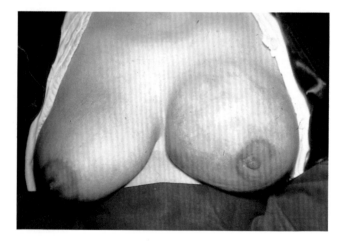

Fig. 4.2 Non-lactating abscess of the left breast.

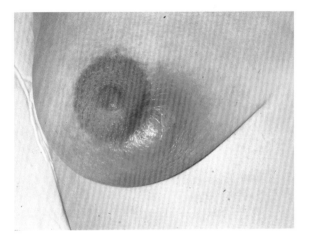

Fig. 4.4 Non-lactating abscess of the right breast.

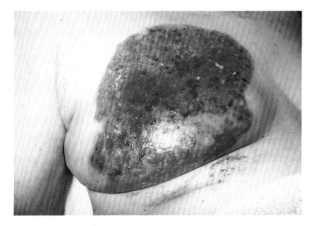

Fig. 6.8 Paget's disease occupying a large area of the breast.

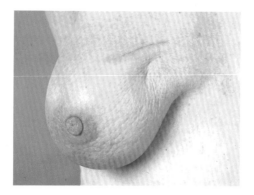

Fig. 7.1 Peau d'orange of the breast.

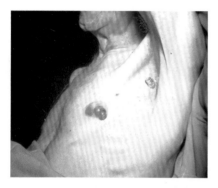

Fig. 7.3 Carcinoma of the male breast. Infiltration of the skin can be seen. The black mark on the skin of the axilla is directly over a palpable and obviously involved axillary node.

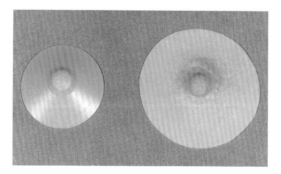

Fig. 8.4 A customized false nipple compared to a commercially obtained one.

SCREENING

Introduction

Screening is the presumptive identification of unrecognized disease by the application of tests, examinations or other procedures which can be applied rapidly. Presumptive is the important word because all screening does is identify two groups of individuals, test positive and test negative. Those who are test positive require a series of diagnostic investigations to determine whether they do truly have the disease being sought, whereas those who are test negative should not need to be further investigated. Screening tests should:

- be simple to apply,
- be cheap,
- be easy to perform,
- be easy and unambiguous to interpret,
- have the ability to define those with disease, and
- exclude those without disease.

Mammography:

- is expensive,
- requires high technology and machinery,
- requires special film and processing,
- requires highly trained radiologists to interpret the films, and
- detects only 95% of all breast cancers at best and only half those lesions detected are malignant.

Mammography is, however, the best screening tool available for the detection of breast cancer and, in fact, is the only screening modality for any malignancy for which the value has been demonstrated by rigorous randomized trials.

Evidence that screening is effective

A number of randomized trials have been undertaken in Europe and the USA and, in addition, there have been a number of non-randomized population-based screening programmes (such as in the UK). There is considerable agreement among trials in showing a reduction in breast cancer mortality between the ages of 50 and 70 (Fig. 5.4). For women over the age of 50 trials indicate an average reduction in mortality of 29%. If one actually estimates the reduction in mortality in those who attend screening then it is estimated that 40% of breast cancer deaths in the attenders can be delayed or prevented. This translates into a 1–2% reduction in overall mortality for women over the age of 50 years.

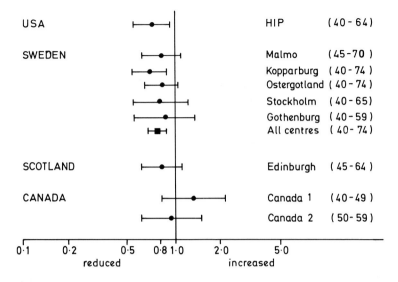

Fig. 5.4 Summary of 7–12 year mortality data in randomized trials of breast cancer screening. The dots represent the absolute reduction in mortality found within each study and the lines emanating from each dot represent the confidence limits. Where the confidence limits do not cross 0, then the reduction in mortality is significant. HIP = Health Insurance Plan.

Compliance, that is the percentage of those invited for screening who attend, is a major factor influencing the effectiveness of screening and as compliance falls so do the benefits of screening.

Characteristics of screen-detected cancers

When compared with patients presenting with symptomatic breast cancers, breast carcinomas detected by screening are more likely to be small, in situ rather than invasive and the invasive cancers are more likely to be better differentiated and of 'special type'. Screen-detected cancers are also more likely to be node negative than symptomatic cancers of the same size (Fig. 5.5). The ability of screening to detect cancers at a very early stage and to influence subsequent mortality indicates that early diagnosis and appropriate treatment of breast cancer reduces the chance of metastatic disease being present.

Overdiagnosis of breast cancer

Some well-differentiated invasive cancers and a number of in situ cancers would almost certainly not have caused symptoms during the

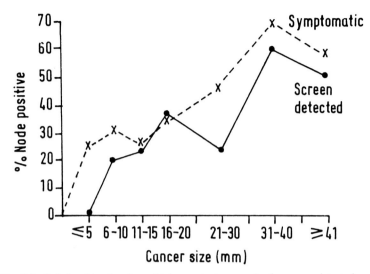

Fig. 5.5   Relationship of node positivity rate to tumour size for screen-detected and symptomatic breast cancers.

patient's lifetime. There are no indications from the currently available data that invasive breast carcinomas are being overdiagnosed by screening. It is possible that a number of cases of in situ carcinoma are detected by screening which would not become clinically significant and this perhaps results in unnecessary treatment in these individuals. Until more is known of the natural history of carcinoma in situ, the extent to which this diagnosis and subsequent over treatment actually occurs during a screening programme remains unknown.

Recommendations for screening

Age range

Current available data indicate that the reduction in mortality is maximal between the age of 50 and 70 years. There is no evidence to support screening in younger women, the major reasons being: the incidence of breast cancer is less frequent in younger women; mammography detects only two-thirds of breast cancers present in women under the age of 50.

Frequency of screening

The most appropriate interval between mammographic screens has yet to be determined. Although from a cost-benefit point of view (cost per year of life gained and cost of quality-adjusted year of life saved) 3-yearly screening of women aged 50–64 years of age appears to be the most cost-effective screening policy, the interval cancer rate climbs rapidly between the second and third year after the initial screen, suggesting that this 3-year interval is too long. In contrast, annual screening is almost certainly too frequent and the optimum frequency for screening is probably 2 years.

Number of mammographic views

Debate continues whether screening by mammography should be by one or two views, but within any National programme such as that within the UK, clear guidelines have been issued and should be adhered to. The current situation in the UK — where the Government states that screening should be by single-view mammography but where more than 40% of units are screening using two views — is unsatisfactory because it leads to confusion amongst both the public and the individuals working in screening units.

Methods of screening

There is no evidence that screening using clinical examination, breast ultrasound or the teaching of breast self examination are effective tools for screening for breast cancer.

Breast self examination. There is evidence that women who perform regular breast self examination detect smaller tumours than those who do not. The problem with breast self examination is that it needs to be taught by experienced personnel and this is costly. Furthermore, only 30–50% of women who are invited to be taught breast self examination attend and little is known of the extent to which women comply and continue to practise breast self examination. Of those studies which have evaluated breast self examination as a screening tool, none has shown a significant reduction in mortality in those women invited to be taught breast self examination. There are also concerns that regular breast self examination induces anxiety amongst women who practise it and results in an increase in the number of benign breast masses detected which then subsequently require assessment.

While women should be encouraged to examine their own breasts and get to know their 'lumps and bumps', it is clear that it is not worthwhile investing money in teaching women regular breast self examination.

Screening of high-risk groups

There are few data to support the regular screening of groups of patients at high risk of breast cancer who are outwith the age range 50–70 years.

Family history

Current recommendations within the USA are that, for women with a first-degree relative who developed premenopausal breast cancer, screening every 2 years should start when the patient is 10 years younger than the age at which the relative developed breast cancer. No consistent policies are applied within the UK.

HRT

The consensus view is that women do not require mammography prior to starting HRT and they should not have screening which starts at a younger age or be screened more regularly than is currently available with the Government screening programme. All women should, however, have a full clinical examination before treatment with HRT is instituted.

Patients with atypical hyerplasia

Current recommendations are that these women should be screened every 2 years.

Genetic screening

It appears that 1–6% of patients with breast cancer have a genetic abnormality on the long arm of chromosome 17; this figure increases to 4–20% in women who develop breast cancer under the age of 45. Within the next few years it will be possible to screen those women who have an affected first-degree relative with breast cancer and identify those individuals with an abnormal gene who are, therefore, at very high risk of developing subsequent breast cancers. How to counsel these patients and how they should be subsequently managed are issues that are currently being debated.

PREVENTION OF BREAST CANCER

The idea that the incidence of breast cancer might be reduced by intervention is not new. Hormonal manipulation by means of oophorectomy was proposed in the 1930s but did not gain favour! More recently the observation that, during trials of tamoxifen as adjuvant treatment for breast cancer, the observed number of second breast cancers was less than expected indicated that this agent might be used to reduce breast cancer incidence. There is a proposal for a study to compare tamoxifen with placebo in ladies (not patients) with risk factors for development of breast cancer which has just received the final go ahead in the UK.

Other measures that have been proposed to reduce the incidence of breast cancer include reduction of dietary fat intake. This would be difficult to achieve without major socio-cultural changes and would probably be opposed by some groups of food producers.

The retinoids are an interesting group of compounds which have effects on the growth and differentiation of epithelial cells. There is both in vivo and in vitro experimental work which suggests that they may have a role in cancer prevention, and a clinical trial of one of the retinoid family is under way.

Other possible preventative agents include selenium, which has not yet been subject to controlled trials.

When considering trials of cancer prevention one has to take account of the number of subjects needed to demonstrate an effect and the type of prevention being planned. Individuals have different risks depending on the extent of their family history of breast cancer and the nature of any previous breast disease. Thus to detect a reduction in relative risk from 3.0 (as might be expected in those at risk with a strong family history) to 2.5 a sample size of approximately 100 000 would be needed; whereas if the intervention reduced the risk to 1.5 then the sample would only need to be around 9500.

A recent report from Guy's hospital has suggested that there is a benefit from operating on patients with breast cancer in the second half of their menstrual cycle. During the first half of the cycle there is a phase of unopposed oestrogen, and experimental work with mice has shown that operating during this phase leads to diminished survival. This retrospective study has been repeated in various centres with conflicting results. Many find no effect at all, others find a significant result in the opposite direction. Since the size of the effect is potentially so great that it would outweigh the benefits of chemotherapy a prospective study has been set up and is currently recruiting patients.

6. Pathology, prognosis, diagnosis and treatment

PATHOLOGY OF BREAST CANCER

Breast cancer arises in the terminal duct lobular unit. Breast cancer was originally described according to its macroscopic appearances and words like scirrhous (meaning woody) still unfortunately appear in the literature. More recently breast cancer has been classified according to histological features; the modern classification is shown in Table 6.1. The division into invasive ductal and invasive lobular types is unfortunate as it is clear that cancers arise in the terminal duct lobular unit (rather than ductal carcinomas arising in the ducts and lobular carcinomas in the lobules). As the terms 'invasive ductal' and 'lobular' are in common usage we continue to refer to them. A more logical classification is into special and no special type (NST) as different prognoses are seen. Many of the special types have a better prognosis.

Invasive carcinoma of NST — frequently called invasive ductal carcinoma — is the most common type accounting for up to 85% of all breast cancers. Special types include invasive lobular carcinoma (classical and variants), invasive tubular, cribriform, medullary and mucinous, with other types being uncommon.

Carcinoma cells confined to within the terminal duct lobular unit and the adjacent ducts, but which have not yet invaded through the basement membrane, are known as carcinoma in situ. As with invasive disease, two main types have been described — ductal carcinoma in situ (DCIS) and lobular carcinoma in situ (LCIS) (Table 6.1). Certain types of DCIS are associated with characteristic microcalcifications giving rise to a typical mammographic pattern. Comedo DCIS is the type of DCIS most likely to be associated with microcalcifications and is often localized, whilst the cribriform and micropapillary type tends to be multifocal. Some authors prefer to classify DCIS as large cell or small cell type (in a similar manner to lung cancer). Whereas LCIS tends to occur in pure form, DCIS often occurs as a mixture of the different types — comedo, cribriform, (micro)papillary and solid. Many more patients

Table 6.1 Histological classification of breast cancer and frequency of presentation in a symptomatic population

History	% frequency
Non-invasive	
Ductal carcinoma in situ	6
Lobular carcinoma in situ	0.2
Invasive	
No special type, 'ductal carcinoma'	68
Special types	
Lobular	
classical	3
variants	7
Tubular	3
Cribriform	3
Medullary	3
Mucinous	2
Microinvasive	2
Papillary	1
Other rare types*	1.8

* includes a few pure apocrine cancers, metaplastic cancers and adenoidcystic cancers

with DCIS are now being diagnosed as the National Breast Screening Programme becomes fully operational.

Invasive ductal carcinomas surrounded by an extensive intraduct component (EIC) are more likely to be multifocal and to need much wider excision in order to achieve clear resection margins.

The breast may be the site of secondaries from other malignancies (such as a lymphoma); these patients require different assessment and treatment and will not be discussed further.

For further details of these histological subtypes and their characteristic features a specialist text book on breast pathology should be consulted (see Further reading).

Handling of the specimen

The pathologist should receive the specimen as soon as possible after surgery — in centres where research is undertaken fresh tissue is taken for study. Routine specimens are fixed in a formalin-containing solution prior to trimming and embedding in paraffin wax. These blocks are then cut with a microtome and stained to allow cellullar detail to be examined. Sections should be taken of the main specimen, resection margins and 'normal' non-involved tissue. The edges of a lumpectomy specimen may be painted with Indian ink to allow assessment of whether the resection margins are involved.

If the specimen is a mastectomy then sections of skin and nipple are also examined. If an axillary dissection is included then the nodes need to be carefully removed and examined individually. This takes time and skill but is important as decisions on adjuvant treatment are based on the result. The number of nodes reported to have been retrieved is often more a function of the pathologist than the surgeon!

Routine reporting

The pathologist is in the best position to give the size of the lesion — clinical estimation is inaccurate although ultrasound can be used to reduce the error. Size is an important prognostic factor and coupled with nodal status and grade can be used to form a prognostic index.

The tumour is assessed for grade using a technique known as Bloom and Richardson grading, named after the first two authors who described it. It is referred to as Scarff-Bloom grading on the Continent and has been modified since its original description. Its use was initially resisted as inter-observer variation was high but it has now been standardized and is very reproducible. The grades are I to III and are made up of three components which are each numerically scored out of 3. These are tubular differentiation, nuclear pleomorphism and the number of mitotic figures present. The higher the score the less well differentiated the tumour. The scores are summated to give a possible range of 3 to 9. Tumours with a score of 3, 4 or 5 are grade I; 6 and 7 grade II; and those scoring 8 and 9 are grade III. Grade alone is an important independent indicator of survival with 85% of patients with a grade I tumour being alive and well at 5 years compared to only a 45% 5-year survival in patients with a grade III lesion. This grading system is designed for use with carcinomas of NST (ductal carcinomas) and should not be used for lobular lesions which are described as low or high grade.

Vascular and lymphatic invasion by tumour can be assessed and is a poor prognostic sign if present. The presence of a round-cell infiltrate into the tumour edge is also assessed but gives less useful information as does the degree of elastosis.

The presence of EIC in an invasive cancer (defined as present if >25% of the main tumour mass is DCIS and if DCIS is present elsewhere in the surrounding tissue) is sought. Many would regard a report of EIC in the original excision specimen as an indication for further excision or a mastectomy if there was a report of EIC in the original biopsy or wide local excision specimen.

Nodal status is of paramount importance and is the gold standard against which other prognostic factors are compared and by which newer factors are judged. A discussion of the clinical importance of nodal status is given in the section on treatment of breast cancer. The pathologist not only has to dissect out the nodes but also examine them carefully. Tumour may only be present in small areas such as the subcapsular space, and it takes time to find these areas. Attempts to improve this process by using a panel of monoclonal antibodies to stain these microdeposits have been tried. They reduce the time that the pathologist needs to spend at the microscope but at the expense of extra preparation and technician time. These techniques do allow more accurate definition of nodal status and identify some patients who would have been classified as node negative as, in fact, being node positive.

Special tests

Specialist tests such as oestrogen receptor, progesterone receptor and other putative histochemical markers of prognosis may be assayed. These are increasingly been performed by immunohistochemical techniques using specific monoclonal antibodies raised against the epitope of interest. Examples of these tests are:

- Oestrogen receptor
- Progesterone receptor
- Epidermal growth factor receptor
- Ki-67
- erb-B2
- Cathepsin D
- nm23

Although most of them are of research interest, their introduction may allow identification of subgroups of patients who either require no adjuvant treatment or need a more aggressive approach.

Some breast neoplasms do not fall into the clear diagnostic groups considered earlier and special tests to determine their nature may be needed. These include special histological stains and the use of monoclonal antibodies.

PROGNOSTIC FACTORS

Survival of patients with breast cancer depends on two different groups of factors: tumour stage, reflecting chronology (i.e. how long the tumour has been present); and biological factors representing the biology or aggressiveness of the tumour.

The search for differential characteristics that allow one to determine a patient's outcome has been the subject of much research. As 50% of women with early breast cancer will be cured by surgery alone or in combination with radiotherapy there is a need to define these patients in order to spare them further therapy. Many factors have been proposed

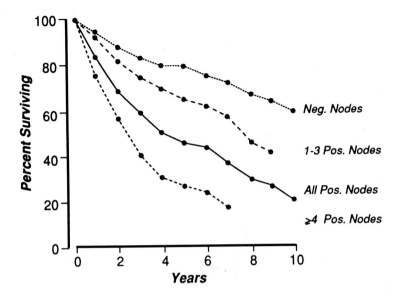

Fig. 6.1   Patients survival in relation to the number of axillary nodes involved.

but few have stood the test of time or rigorous analysis. What works for one set of patients often fails to transfer to a different cohort. The criteria for a prognostic factor to be clinically accepted has been outlined by Dr McGuire. The factor must:

• have biological relevance,
• be reproducible in different laboratories,
• be validated prospectively in a large series of patients, and
• be confirmed independently by other workers.

In addition, they must have an appropriate cut-off point; must identify a population at high (or low) risk (there also needs to be an appropriate therapy which this population can be offered); and, ideally, they should be cheap and give an answer quickly. Many candidates have been proposed for prognostic factors and these are listed under Special tests (see page 94).

Prognostic factors may be divided into those obtained routinely (such as size, grade, nodal status) and those needing special biochemical or immunohistochemical tests.

Nodal status

The single 'gold standard' against which all other factors should be compared is nodal status. The more nodes involved the worse the prognosis (Fig. 6.1) with an average 10-year survival of 60–70% for node-negative patients dropping to 20–30% for those with involved nodes; adjuvant chemotherapy is now routinely given to premenopausal women in this group. There are probably subgroups of high-risk node-negative patients who would also benefit from adjuvant chemotherapy.

Histology

Overall tumours of certain special type (classical lobular, tubular, cribriform, medullary, mucinous and papillary) have a much better prognosis than tumours of NST. This association appears independent of grade. Invasive carcinoma of tubular and cribriform types are associated with an excellent long-term survival and few patients with these tumours die as a result of their disease. Invasive medullary carcinomas are unusual tumours in that according to the Bloom and Richardson classification they are grade III and yet they are associated with a very much better prognosis than grade III NST carcinomas. In a series of patients from Edinburgh the 5-year survival for patients with tumours of these special types was 91% compared with 47% for carcinomas of NST. Of patients alive 20 years after treatment for breast cancer, over 40% of long-term survivors had tumours of these special types which is more than twice the percentage (15%) of all breast cancers which are of these types.

Size

Size is a crude predictor of the metastatic potential of a tumour — larger tumours having a slightly higher incidence of metastasis to the regional nodes. Even small tumours may have nodal involvement (about 17% of those tumours smaller than 1 cm are node positive) but generally most women with tumours measuring less than 1cm and negative nodes have an excellent prognosis.

Tumour grade

Tumour grade as assessed by the Bloom and Richardson system has the ability to predict outcome with 86% of patients with grade I tumours being alive at 5 years compared to 57% of those with a grade III lesion.

These three factors may be combined to form a prognostic index which allows greater separation of survival curves. The best known of these indices is that defined by the Nottingham group based on a retrospective multivariate analysis of many hundred cases where survival and time to relapse was well quantified (Nottingham Prognostic Index; NPI). They combined tumour grade, nodal status and size in the formula:

$$NPI = (0.2 \times \text{size cm}) + \text{grade} + \text{stage}$$

to give a figure. Grade was assessed by the Bloom and Richardson method and scored 1 to 3. Stage was based on nodal status and was the combination of a triple-node biopsy (the low axilla, high axilla and internal mammary chain). They have shown this index works in a second, prospectively collected, cohort and use it routinely to determine which patients need no further treatment after excision and radiotherapy. This index has been shown to be reproducible and even to work in Yorkshire (Fig. 6.2)! In Nottingham the tumours were all graded by one pathologist whereas in Yorkshire they were graded by a number of pathologists suggesting that grading is not as difficult as was once suggested. The Yorkshire surgeons adopted a more pragmatic approach to assessing nodes and did not (like most centres) perform internal mammary sampling.

Newer biological factors

Other factors related to the biology of the tumour have been described. There are problems with standardization and inter-laboratory variation for many. Quality Assurance schemes have been implemented for some of the more important ones under the auspices of groups such as European Organization for Research and Treatment of Cancer (EORTC). In the USA, where much more attention is paid to these factors, commercial assay of multiple factors has become big business. Many are still experimental and further work is needed before their place is established; many are not routinely measured in the UK as treatment decisions are made on the basis of more conventional factors.

Oestrogen receptor (ER)

ER status was the first of the 'biological' markers to be studied. Approximately 60% of tumours contain detectable ER as assessed either biochemically using a radioligand assay or immunocytochemically using a monoclonal antibody raised against an ER-related protein. Its initial promise as a useful discriminent has not held up — there is only a 5–10% difference in disease-free survival between patients with node-negative ER-positive tumours and those with node-negative ER-negative tumours. The survival after first relapse is, however, predicted by ER status with ER-positive patients living longer and having a better response to therapy be it chemotherapy or endocrine treatment.

Progesterone receptor (PR)

PRs have been described and depend upon an intact ER pathway in order to be expressed. Their presence therefore tends to correlate with

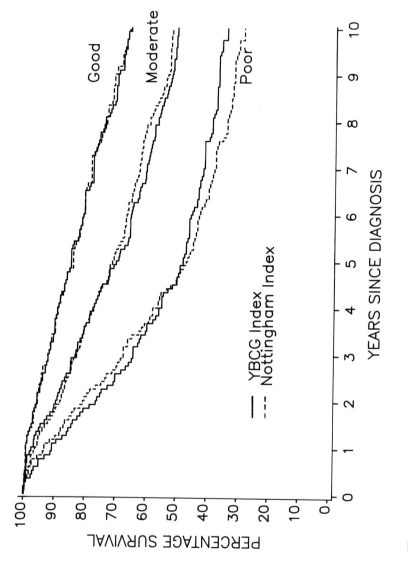

Fig. 6.2   Comparison of the Nottingham and Yorkshire Breast Cancer Group prognostic indices.

ER status but does allow definition of a subgroup of ER-positive patients with a better prognosis.

Cell kinetics and ploidy

Ploidy is a measurement of the relative proportion of DNA in each cell and can be combined with measurements of the rate of cell growth and division. The percentage of cells in active cell division (S-phase) can be determined by flow cytometry. S-phase is a better predictor of relapse and survival than ploidy but both can be used to good effect in the node-negative woman. Diploid tumours have a lower risk of relapse than aneuploid ones and low S-phase tumours have a more favourable prognosis regardless of ploidy. These analyses can be performed in both fresh and paraffin-embedded tissue. The use of the antibody Ki-67 allows an easier estimation of proliferation.

erb-B2

This protein is a cell membrane receptor and is the product of the *neu* oncogene. It has a similarity to epidermal growth factor receptor and can be detected in both paraffin-embedded and frozen sections by immunohistochemistry. There are problems in deciding whether a tumour should be classified as positive or negative. Node-positive women (already candidates for adjuvant therapy) with increased expression of erb-B2 fare less well; but the situation is less clear for those with node-negative tumours. erb-B2 has been used in conjunction with other prognostic factors and generally in each subset those with erb-B2-positive tumours have a worse outcome.

Epidermal growth factor receptor (EGFr)

This is another cell membrane protein which is related to an oncogene product (v-erb-B — originally named after the erythroblastic virus which caused cancer in chickens). Binding of its ligand (EGF) promotes growth of cancer cells including breast cancer cells grown in culture. The presence of EGFrs correlates with other prognostic factors and there is a relationship between its presence and high grade (Bloom and Richardson grade III) and other indicators of poor outlook. EGFr does not correlate with nodal status and can be used to divide node-negative patients into two groups with good separation of survival curves. It has been added to the Nottingham prognostic index to increase its power. It has also been correlated directly with survival and is a predictor of a reduced disease-free and overall survival. EGFr also correlates with response to endocrine therapy — elderly patients treated with tamoxifen

alone were five times more likely to respond if their tumours were
EGFr negative.

Cathepsin D

This is one member of a family of proteases whose activity is stimulated
by oestrogens. It may contribute to metastasis by dissolving basement
membrane and extracellular matrix thus allowing cancer cells to spread.
There is a good correlation between presence of cathepsin D and
prognosis with some studies showing that patients with low levels of
cathepsin D and positive nodes actually outlived those with negative
nodes and high levels of cathepsin D.

p53

This is the product of a nuclear oncogene and is coded on the short arm
of chromosome 17. It appears to be responsible for preventing cellular
division in an uncontrolled fashion. As such it works by stabilizing the
cell and abnormalities might be expected to allow uncontrolled growth.
The protein occurs both as a wild type and as a mutant. Care has to be
taken in using an appropriate antibody as the protein is unstable. It
seems that a group of patients who have a greatly increased risk of
breast, ovarian and bowel cancer (the Li-Fraumeni syndrome) have an
abnormality of their p53 expression.

Other factors

Heat shock protein, the antimetastatic gene nm23, pS2, laminin receptors, IGF-I receptors and somatostatin receptors are amongst other
factors studied. They are not yet in common usage.

Use of prognostic factors

Patients can be categorized into good or bad prognostic groups on the
results of the above factors. They allow definition of a subgroup of
node-negative patients whose outlook is so good that no further
(adjuvant) treatment is needed and a group of node-positive high-risk
patients whose prognosis is so poor that intensive measures such as
high-dose chemotherapy and bone marrow transplantation might be
considered. It is rare that anyone has all the characteristics of the good
or bad group and the relative merits of each factor needs to be considered
before deciding what treatment is appropriate.

DIAGNOSIS OF BREAST CANCER

The majority of patients with breast cancer still present with a breast lump, although it is hoped that the number of patients with impalpable cancers will increase as the Screening Programme should permit earlier identification of breast cancers in the numerically important 50–65-year-old age group. A definite diagnosis should be on all breast lumps and it should not be assumed that a lump is benign because the mammography or cytology are inconclusive. All patients should have a tissue diagnosis prior to proceeding to definite surgery. This is increasingly made by cytology rather than open biopsy although the latter may still be necessary on occasions. The combination of clinical examination, mammography and fine needle cytology (the triple approach) allows a definitive diagnosis to be made and a treatment plan to be formulated.

If the patient attends a specialist breast clinic the diagnosis may well be established at the time of their first visit. This has considerable advantages in that the news can be broken without a long wait and treatments can be discussed. It is appropriate to have a breast nurse specialist/counsellor present when the diagnosis is given as she will be able to reiterate and reinforce the information passed to the patient as well as acting as a channel for support. A date for staging, surgery (or other primary therapy) can be planned and arrangements for a home visit made. A planned delay of 5–10 days from diagnosis to treatment is often helpful to the patient and her relatives and allows for the home visit (unfortunately not widely available as yet) or further discussions as appropriate.

Patients referred from the screening service may have a diagnosis of malignancy made on cytology either by needling of a suspicious area or by stereolocalization of an impalpable lesion. They often need extra care and counselling as they were essentially well women until they attended for mammography. These women are often more anxious by the time they are assessed despite the probability that any lesion picked up at screening is likely to be of better prognosis.

Staging

Once a breast cancer has been diagnosed the patient is staged. The general staging classifications for cancers are not particularly well suited for breast cancer but, as there is no agreement on a better one, the Tumour size-Node-Metastasis (TNM) classification is used. The older UICC stagings are also still in usage but the modern classification of staging and the correlation with TNM is given in Table 6.2. There is confusion between clinical and pathological staging — tumour size and nodal status often change when the definitive histological report is

Table 6.2   TNM classification and relationship to stage

T_{1s}	in situ
T_1	< 2 cm (T_{1a} ⩽ 0.5 cm, T_{1b} > 0.5–1.0 cm, T_{1c} > 1 cm ⩽ 2.0 cm)
T_2	> 2–5 cm
T_3	> 5 cm
T_{4a}	Involvement of chest wall
b	Involvement of skin (includes ulceration, direct infiltration, peau d'orange and satellite nodules)
c	a and b together
d	inflammatory cancer
N_0	No regional node metastasis
N_1	Mobile ipsilateral nodes
N_2	Fixed ipsilateral nodes
N_3	Internal mammary node involvement (rarely clinically detectable)
M_0	No evidence of metastasis
M_1	Distant metastasis (includes ipsilateral supraclavicular nodes)

Correlation of UICC (1987) stage and TNM		
Stage I	=	T_1, N_0, M_0
Stage II	=	T_1, N_1, M_0
		T_2, N_{0-1}, M_0
Stage III	=	any T, N_2 or T_3, N_1, M_0 or
		T_4, N_{0-2}, M_0
Stage IV	=	any T, any N, M_1

Table 6.3   Use of staging investigations

Stage	Investigation
I	Full blood count
	Liver function tests
	Chest X-ray
II	As above but may need liver or bone scan if in clinical trials
III	As above but with calcium phosphate measurement, liver and bone scans
IV	As stage III

available. The TNM system was designed to be used clinically and should be reserved for this.

There is a low incidence of detectable metastatic disease for patients with stage 1 ($T_1 N_0$) tumours and in the absence of hepatomegaly or bone pain scans of liver and bone have been shown to be worthless. Investigations should include a full blood count, liver function tests and a chest X-ray. For those with bigger or more advanced tumours bone and liver scans may be ordered if their outcome is going to change clinical management (Table 6.3).

Patients with recurrent disease need full staging prior to treatment

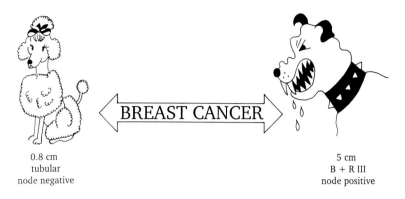

0.8 cm
tubular
node negative

5 cm
B + R III
node positive

Fig. 6.3 A cartoon of an explanation of the biology of breast cancers. Comparing breast cancer to a dog allows visualization of a range of behaviours. B + R III = Bloom and Richardson Grade III carcinoma.

(liver ultrasound and bone scan plus a chest X-ray) in order to identify metastatic sites and tumour load.

Attempts to look for micrometastatic disease have included bone marrow aspiration and radioisotope-labelled antibody studies. The former undoubtedly allows detection of cancer cells in the marrow and some groups show this to adversely affect the prognosis whereas the latter has proved disappointing and needs further refinement.

The use of carcinoembryonic antigen (CEA) measurement either alone or in combination with erythrocyte sedimentation rate (ESR) and CA-125 has been advocated by some but has low specificity and sensitivity.

Once the patient has been staged decisions have to be made about appropriate therapy. The alternatives should be discussed with the patient and they should be encouraged to participate in decisions. One tool we have found useful in talking through the biology of breast cancer with our patients is to compare breast cancer to a dog. Depending on the stage or prognostic factors the patient can then be placed on a scale that ranges from a rottweiler (i.e. a 5 cm Bloom and Richardson grade III lesion with more than 10 nodes positive) to a poodle (0.8 cm screen-detected node-negative tubular cancer) (Fig. 6.3). This allows the patient and relatives to visualize their disease — it obviously works as many patients ask if theirs was a rottweiler when the results are being discussed. Other methods of helping patients come to terms with their diagnosis include taping the 'bad news' consultation and giving the patient the tape to take home. This subject is discussed further in section 4.

TREATMENT OF BREAST CANCER

Introduction

Discussions of the management of breast cancer traditionally divide the subject into early and advanced categories. This was based on the criteria of operability with 'early' usually encompassing stages I and II and advanced being stages III and IV disease. The use of 'early' is a misnomer as true early breast cancer would be too small to detect clinically, as once a tumour is palpable, micrometastatic disease is probable. Early should refer to the biology of the tumour — some patients present with large ulcerated cancers that have been present for a long time and yet they have no evidence of metastases whilst some present with metastatic disease with a very small primary (and some without a detectable lesion at all).

The treatment of the patient with 'early' breast cancer has two main aims — to achieve local disease control and to treat any micrometastatic disease. Although breast cancer is often a systemic disease at presentation there are many patients who are cured by primary surgery (with or without radiotherapy) alone. Deciding which patients need further therapy has recently been simplified but many questions remain to be answered.

Treatment of non-invasive breast cancer

Ductal carcinoma in situ (DCIS)

The 'correct' treatment of DCIS is as yet unclear. Most would agree that the area of malignancy needs to be completely excised. (What constitutes clear resection margins is also debated). It is clear that when compared with the general a patient with localized DCIS has nine times the risk of developing invasive breast cancer within the following 15 years. If the area is small and unifocal the patient may be eligible for the United Kingdom Co-ordinating Committee on Cancer Research (UKCCCR) sponsored trial. This randomizes patients to: no further therapy; tamoxifen 20 mg/day for 2 years; radiotherapy alone; or a combination of tamoxifen and radiotherapy. It requires the resection margins to be clear, there to be no evidence of microinvasion, and all microcalcifications to have been removed. These criteria, unfortunately, are difficult to fulfil and recruitment is slow. There has been little enthusiasm for randomization into the radiotherapy arm, but this may change now that a recent study from the USA has shown a significant reduction in the numbers of invasive cancers developing after adding radiotherapy to wide local excision. There is also concern that any answer obtained will apply only to this subgroup of DCIS and may not be applicable to patients with a larger area of DCIS or if microinvasion is present.

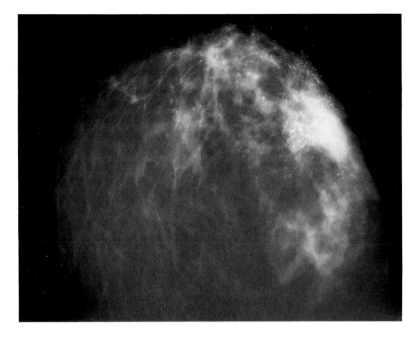

Fig. 6.4   Mammogram showing multifocal DCIS.

If the area is large or multifocal (as judged on mammography) (Fig. 6.4) then a mastectomy is indicated. This could be of the subcutaneous type with immediate placement of a prosthesis if the patient wishes. It is paradoxical that women with invasive breast cancer may receive conservation treatment with lumpectomy and radiotherapy, whereas those with non-invasive disease may be recommended a mastectomy. If a mastectomy is performed it is usual to sample the lower axillary nodes as an occasional positive node is encountered if the DCIS is extensive. An axillary clearance is not necessary.

The risk of DCIS in the other breast is the same as the risk of contralateral breast cancer in patients with invasive disease — about 0.6% per year unlike lobular carcinoma in situ which frequently occurs bilaterally.

Lobular carcinoma in situ (LCIS)

This rarer form of non-invasive breast cancer differs in presentation, biological behaviour and implications for treatment. LCIS does not typically form microcalcifications and is therefore not easily detectable on X-ray and is usually found incidentally on biopsy. It can be found in the contralateral breast in 30% of cases and in the residual breast (if treated by mastectomy) in up to 70% of cases. If LCIS is associated with invasive lobular carcinoma the incidence of nodal involvement is very low and LCIS having been diagnosed by biopsy should be treated by careful follow-up in the expectation of ipsilateral or contralateral disease which may be invasive. This should take the form of clinical examination, annual mammography with ultrasound and biopsy of any area of suspicion.

Treatment of invasive breast cancer

Local control

Local control is important. A recurrence in the mastectomy wound or at the site of a local resection is damaging both oncologically and psychologically. There is debate about whether such a recurrence compromises survival (the majority of reports claim that it does not) but it does require further treatment. The adoption of more conservative surgery might be expected to lead to a higher incidence of recurrence but this can be minimized by achieving clear resection margins and by the subsequent use of radiotherapy as well as by advising patients with large, aggressive tumours to consider mastectomy.

Conservation therapy

Not everyone is suitable for conservation therapy — those with multi-focal disease on clinical examination or mammography or a large, centrally placed tumour are often better off with a mastectomy as the resultant defect is not attractive and it may be impossible to provide a satisfactory prosthesis. These patients can be offered a reconstruction either as a primary or secondary procedure. In some centres primary systemic therapy, usually chemotherapy, is offered to those with large tumours to downstage them and thus allow smaller resections (neoadjuvant chemotherapy).

The aim of achieving local control includes attention to the axilla. There is still a great deal of debate about how the axilla should be managed, and this is addressed later.

Local control is achieved by the use of surgery in the majority of cases (because most patients are still referred to surgeons and because it is often an appropriate modality).

Whilst it is possible to treat even small cancers with chemotherapy and radiotherapy this is time consuming and tends to be reserved for large T_2, T_3 and T_4 lesions. Large doses of radiotherapy are needed in the presence of an intact tumour and cosmesis is poor. For smaller cancers breast conservation is the most common primary treatment. This takes the form of a lumpectomy or wide local excision performed through an appropriate incision to give a good cosmetic result (see Fig. 6.2).

Table 6.4   Indications and contraindications for selection of patients for breast conservation (adapted from NIH Consensus Conference Statement 1991)

Indications	T_1, T_2($\leqslant$4 cm), N_0, N_1, M_0
	T_2 > 4 cm in large breasts
Contraindications	T_3–T_4, N_2 or M_1
	Large or central tumours in small breasts
	Multifocal/multicentric disease
	Collagen vascular disease
Relative contraindications	An extensive in situ component
	Young age (under 35–39 years)
	Widespread lymphatic invasion

Impalpable lesions should be investigated by stereotactic or ultrasound-guided fine needle aspiration cytology (FNAC) as appropriate and Figure 2.19 outlines how this assists in the management of these patients. In units without access to stereotactic aspiration cytology, patients with lesions considered to be suspicious should have these either widely excised or biopsied depending on the degree of suspicion, with any lymph node surgery being performed as a separate procedure.

Patients suitable for breast conservation are listed in Table 6.4 and include:

● those with a single clinical and mammographic lesion measuring 4 cm or less without signs of local advancement (T_1, T_2 < 4 cm), extensive nodal involvement (N_0, N_1) or metastases (M_0); and
● those with tumours bigger than 4 cm and large breasts.

There is no age limit for breast conservation and elderly, fit patients should be treated in the same way as younger patients.

Lesions which are potentially unsuitable for breast conservation are summarized in Table 6.4 and include:

● Patients for whom breast conservation treatment would produce an unacceptable cosmetic result. This includes the majority of central lesions and carcinomas over 4 cm in size; additionally, these larger tumours have been excluded from most prospective studies of breast conservation and so there is little information on the outcome of treating such tumours by conservation. Using primary systemic chemotherapy, however, it is now possible to shrink large tumours to allow breast conserving surgery to be performed. In Milan tumours measuring 3 cm or over are traditionally treated by mastectomy, but in a series of these tumours treated by primary chemotherapy 81% were reduced in size to less than 3 cm and were subsequently suitable for treatment by breast conservation.

- Patients with multiple macroscopic tumour foci treated by breast conservation have a high incidence of local recurrence and are better treated by mastectomy, ideally with immediate breast reconstruction. Although multifocal or multicentric disease may be evident clinically, it is often only identified by mammography.
- Patients with bilateral disease can be treated by bilateral conservation, but bilateral mastectomy with immediate reconstruction is preferred by some.

Certain clinical and pathological factors may influence selection of patients for breast conservation, because of their potential impact on local recurrence after breast conserving therapy. These include young age (< 35–39 years), the presence of extensive DCIS associated with the invasive tumour (EIC) and widespread lymphatic invasion.

As clear resection margins are important to reduce local relapse, care should be taken to widely excise the lesion. The edges should be identified by clips or sutures to allow orientation of the specimen. Some surgeons go on to take cavity shavings — this allows the pathologist to confirm if the resection margins are clear. If tumour is present in the shavings then either further local excision or a mastectomy is indicated. It is clear from the literature that radiotherapy will not always compensate for involved margins. A quadrantectomy (tylectomy) is popular in some countries but is a misnomer in that it is impossible to divide the breast into discrete quadrants. Such excisions aim to get wider margins (3 cm) and are associated with higher rates of local control but much poorer cosmetic outcomes.

Local surgery alone may be sufficient treatment for small areas of DCIS or small invasive tumours of special type. This hypothesis is to be tested in a trial run by the British Association of Surgical Oncology (BASO) where patients with special type and well-differentiated cancers will, after surgery, be randomized to no further treatment, radiotherapy and/or tamoxifen.

Wide local excision of palpable lesions

The aim of this procedure is to remove the palpable lesion with a 1 cm margin of surrounding normal breast tissue. The incision should be placed along Langer's lines (Fig. 6.5) directly over the lesion, and it is inappropriate to use circumareolar incisions for lesions some distance away from the nipple; the reason for this is that if re-excision is required this procedure is almost impossible through such an incision. Removal of skin overlying the lesion is unnecessary unless the lesion is very superficial. The cosmetic result after breast conserving surgery is influenced by the amount of skin excised, poor results being obtained in

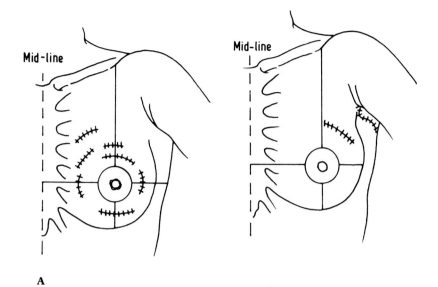

A

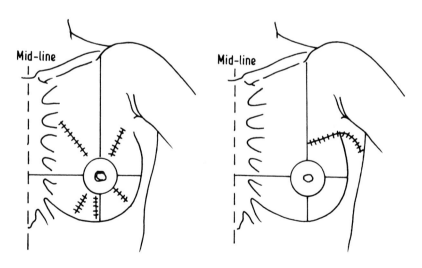

B

Fig. 6.5 Recommended (**A**) and non-recommended (**B**) incisions for breast conserving surgery.

those who have had a large amount of skin removed. If the patient has had a previous incomplete excision, then the previous scar should be excised. Having made the skin incision, the fingers of the left hand are placed over the lesion and dissection is performed 1 cm beyond the fingertips so that the line of incision through the breast tissue is beyond the limit of the carcinoma. Although in superficial lesions it is sometimes necessary to dissect in the plane between the breast tissue and subcutaneous fat, skin flaps should not be undermined by dissecting into the subcutaneous fat, as thin skin flaps are associated with a poor postoperative cosmetic appearance. Dissection is usually continued through the breast down to the pectoral fascia with no attempt being made to excise this fascia, unless it is tethered to the tumour or the tumour is directly involving it. Where the carcinoma infiltrates the muscle, a fillet of muscle should be removed, the aim being to gain a rim of normal tissue around the tumour. Having reached the pectoral fascia, the breast is elevated from this fascia, the lesion grasped between fingers and thumb and excision completed at the other margins. In superficial lesions an adequate excision can usually be performed without excising a full thickness portion of breast tissue down to pectoral fascia. Specimens should be orientated prior to submission to a pathologist with sutures or ligaclips. Meticulous haemostasis is secured with diathermy, the cavity is lavaged with diluted savlon left in situ for 2 min. Savlon (dilute chlorhexadine) has been shown to be tumoricidal at this concentration and within this time period.

Stereotactic wide local excision

Impalpable lesions are localized prior to surgery as discussed earlier for needle localization biopsy. Using the mammograms as a guide, a block of tissue 1–2 cm around the mammographic lesion is excised. The specimen is orientated with ligaclips and then X-rayed. The radiograph of the excised specimen is inspected during the operation, and having orientated the specimen with ligaclips, it is possible to assess the completeness of excision; if the lesion approaches any resection margin, further tissue can be excised and orientated from the appropriate area. Using this technique it is possible to achieve complete excision in over 80% of both invasive and in situ carcinomas. Wound management after the lesion has been excised is as for wide local excision.

Postoperative radiotherapy

Radiotherapy services are provided on a regional or sub-regional basis and patients may have to travel long distances for this treatment. Commonly the radiation is given using a linear accelerator to deliver

Table 6.5 Relationship between age and local recurrence rates at 5 years following breast conserving treatment

Age	Local recurrence rate
⩽ 35	17%
35–50	12%
⩾ 51	6%

high energy X-rays with 40–50 Gy (equivalent to 4000–5000 rad) being given to the breast over 4 weeks in daily fractions of 180–200 cGY. Some centres prescribe higher doses and the dose per fraction may also vary. A top-up or boost (15–20 Gy) to the excision site can be given by further external beam irradiation or by the use of radioactive implants. These may be iridium wires which are inserted around the tumour site. Precise indications for boosting and technique are not well defined.

The survival rates after lumpectomy are equivalent to those after more radical surgery, and the former is now the treatment of choice for appropriate patients. The swing away from mastectomy as the routine operation for patients with breast cancer is to be welcomed but must not become a goal in its own right — the interests of some patients will be compromised if the only operation offered is a lumpectomy.

The axilla will be irradiated if it has not been treated by surgery and the ipsilateral supraclavicular fossa may also be treated if the axillary nodes were involved. The addition of radiotherapy to lumpectomy reduced the local recurrence rate from 39% to 10% in the National Surgical Adjuvant Breast Project B-06 (NSABP B-06) (see Chapter 9) and reductions from 25% to 5% are quoted in other studies.

Risk factors for local recurrence after breast conservation

Large variations have been reported (2–22% at 5 years) from different centres in rates of recurrence within the treated breast following breast conservation therapy for invasive breast carcinoma.

Patient-related factors

Rates of local recurrence appear to correlate closely with age, being more frequent in younger patients. In women under the age of 35 the risk of local recurrence is approximately three times the risk of patients over the age of 50 (Table 6.5). A single study has indicated that breast recurrence is less frequent in women with large breasts, whether this relates to it being possible to perform more generous excisions in these patients is unknown.

Tumour-related factors

Tumour location, size, the presence of skin or nipple retraction and the presence or absence of axillary nodal involvement have not been consistently shown to be factors predictive of recurrence within the breast following conservation therapy. Local failure rates appear to relate to:
The completeness of excision. If the pathologist reports the presence of invasive or in situ cancer at the margins of the excision, then local recurrence is approximately three times more likely to occur than if the margins are reported to be clear.
The presence of an extensive in situ component (EIC). If 25% of the tumour mass is composed of in situ carcinoma, and in situ carcinoma is also present in the tissue surrounding the tumour, then the carcinoma is considered to have an EIC. Patients who have a tumour which is EIC positive have approximately three times the risk of local recurrence when compared to patients whose tumours are EIC negative.
Lymphatic/vascular invasion. If the pathologist reports the presence of tumour within vascular or lymphatic channels within or around the invasive cancer, then breast recurrence is approximately twice as common as tumours where this feature is absent.

Treatment-related factors

As outlined above the completeness of excision is a major factor predicting local recurrence. Both the completeness of excision and the amount of normal tissue removed around the carcinoma appear related to local disease control — the wider the margins the lower the rate of local recurrence. The volume of normal tissue excised is particularly important in tumours which are EIC positive. In these cancers a very wide excision is necessary to gain adequate local control rates.
Radiotherapy, chemotherapy and tamoxifen all reduce local relapse rates after breast conserving therapy. Radiotherapy is routinely used as part of breast conserving therapy because of its clear reduction in local recurrence rates. The interval between surgery and radiotherapy may be important and there are suggestions that the rate of local recurrence increases if radiotherapy is delayed. There is some evidence to suggest that increased doses of radiotherapy improve local control rates, but the higher the dose of radiotherapy given, the poorer the overall cosmetic result. There is thus a delicate balance between achieving adequate local control rates and satisfactory cosmetic results (Fig. 6.6).

Significance and treatment of local recurrence

An isolated breast recurrence does not appear to be a threat to survival, although breast recurrence is a predictor of distant disease which should

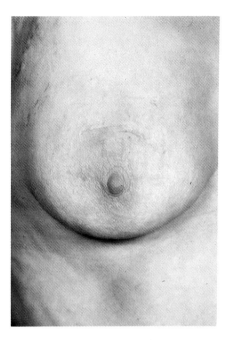

Fig. 6.6 Cosmetic result following conservation therapy.

be sought in all patients presenting with an apparently isolated breast recurrence. Isolated recurrences can be treated by re-excision or mastectomy. Although it is known that re-excision is associated with a high rate of further recurrence, if the initial recurrence occurs more than 5 years after surgery, and the margins of the re-excision are clear of disease, adequate long-term control can be achieved. For local recurrences not fulfilling these criteria, mastectomy is indicated unless the local recurrence is associated with metastatic disease when systemic therapy is required. Uncontrollable local recurrence is uncommon after breast conservation but does occur and is difficult to treat.

Diagnosis of a recurrence after previous local excision and radiotherapy is not always straightforward and there may be a delay in achieving a diagnosis. Cytology can be misleading and mammography difficult to interpret.

The criteria for conservation therapy are shown in Table 6.4.

PRIMARY MEDICAL THERAPY

This is increasingly being used for larger operable breast cancers. Induction (neoadjuvant) chemotherapy has been shown in Milan to

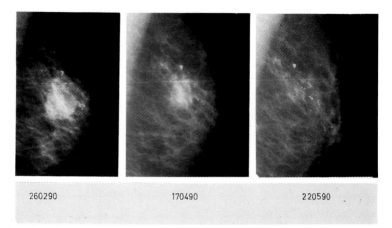

260290   170490   220590

Fig. 6.7 Three mammograms from a patient undergoing primary medical treatment showing disappearance of the tumour mass. Note that the microcalcifications remain.

shrink large T_2 and T_3 tumours and thus allow quadrantectomy rather than mastectomy. Figure 6.7 shows the mammograms of a patient with a large breast cancer receiving combination chemotherapy. The tumour mass can clearly be seen to have disappeared although the microcalcifications remain. Failure to proceed to some form of additional treatment (usually surgery) will lead to local relapse. It is not yet known whether patients who achieve a complete clinical response can be further managed by radiotherapy alone. The surgery may be difficult as there may be little to feel on dissection and a localizing wire may be neccessary.

MASTECTOMY

Historically, mastectomy has been the treatment of choice for breast cancer as the prevalent hypothesis was of a centrifugal spread. The lymph nodes were supposed to act as filters with secondary spread occurring only when their capacity was exhausted. It therefore seemed logical to perform ever more 'heroic' (extensive) surgery in an attempt to get beyond the growing edge of the tumour. This dogma, based on the studies of Handley, held sway for 100 years and was championed by Halsted whose name is still attached to a radical mastectomy. In the 1920s some American surgeons went so far as to perform forequarter amputations in an attempt to clear the disease.

A mastectomy is now taken to be an operation that removes the breast tissue with some overlying skin (including the nipple). This is termed a total mastectomy. If the skin and nipple are left intact and the breast tissue removed the operation is termed a subcutaneous mastectomy. A radical mastectomy includes removal of the pectoralis muscles and the axillary contents. This was modified by Patey (modified radical mastectomy) who left the pectoralis major muscle but divided pectoralis minor which still allowed the axilla to be cleared. The most common breast resecting operation in this country is the total mastectomy combined with a limited axillary dissection or sampling ('simple mastectomy') or with a full axillary clearance ('modified radical mastectomy'). The range of resective breast surgery is as follows:

- None
- Incision biopsy
- Excision biopsy
- Wide local excision
- Segmental excision (segmentectomy)
- Quadrantectomy (tylectomy)
- Subcutaneous mastectomy
- Total mastectomy
- Modified radical mastectomy
- Radical mastectomy

Technique

The incisions are planned to allow skin flaps to be created which will close neatly but without undue tension. They should be of equal length to prevent 'dog ears' in the final scar. Dissection is performed under the flaps until the fascia covering the pectoralis muscles is reached. Breast tissue is then elevated from the fascia and removed. Haemostasis is achieved with ties or diathermy, and low pressure suction drains are inserted under the skin to remove serosanguinous exudate and to allow the flaps to stick to the chest wall. The wound is closed with subcutaneous and subcuticular sutures such as polydioxone sulphate (Ethicon) or Maxon (Davis and Geck). No formal dressing is required although Steri-strips applied to the length of the wound and then crossways across it reduce any wound edge oedema and give a neater final scar. The patient begins arm exercises, taught preoperatively, on the day after surgery and the drains are removed when the drainage is less then 50 ml. The length of time they drain depends on the extent of axillary surgery.

Complications after mastectomy

These include: seroma; infection; flap necrosis; and lymphoedema.

Seroma

These occur in the dead space under the flaps and are caused by the transudation of fluid across the large surface area where the breast and lymphatics once were. Suction drainage has been shown in several trials to be effective in reducing significant seromas as well as reducing the incidence of wound infection. They should be of low pressure as high pressure suction merely collapses skin around the drain and blocks it.

Infection

This is generally secondary to tissue necrosis caused by cutting the flaps too thin which results in devascularization. Prophylactic antibiotics are not indicated unless for some other underlying reason such as the insertion of a tissue expander or prostheses — good surgical technique is more important.

Flap necrosis

Again this is usually as a result of technical shortcomings secondary to devascularization of the flaps.

Lymphoedema

This is uncommon after a simple mastectomy and its incidence rises with the amount of axillary surgery performed. The combination of extensive axillary surgery and radiotherapy gives a high incidence of lymphoedema and should be avoided. When it occurs, compression therapy either by means of a mechanical sleeve (as provided with a Flowtron machine) or by regular bandaging is needed. The latter is more time-consuming and requires considerable skill, but is probably more effective in reducing the oedema. After active therapy the arm is placed in an elasticated compression sleeve. This should be measured on an individual basis for each patient.

Other complications

These are rare but include pneumothorax and injury to neurovascular structures.

Radiotherapy after mastectomy

The question of whether chest wall irradiation is indicated after mastectomy was controversial, but its role has been better defined. Studies by McWhirter in Edinburgh showed that simple mastectomy and radiotherapy was as effective a treatment as radical mastectomy in terms of both disease control and survival. The more recent Cancer Research Campaign (CRC) trial, where 2800 women with stage I and II breast cancer were randomized to receive radiotherapy or no radiotherapy after mastectomy, showed no difference in survival but demonstrated a marked improvement in local control rates for those receiving radiotherapy. Those not having radiotherapy had approximately three times the risk of local recurrence, the majority of which (but not all) were controllable by radiotherapy given at the time of relapse. At one time radiotherapy was standard treatment after all mastectomies but there is now a move to a more selective policy. The indications for radiotherapy postmastectomy are:

- large tumours (> 4 cm);
- high-grade tumours (Bloom and Richardson grade III);
- node-positive tumours (> 4), especially if extranodal disease is seen; and
- node-negative tumours with widespread vascular/lymphatic invasion.

Those in the remaining group who go on to develop local recurrence can be treated at that time in the knowledge that, in the majority, disease will be controlled by this treatment.

THE AXILLA

Introduction

This subject, more than any other, causes heated debate. The options for axillary treatment range from nothing through sampling and limited axillary dissection, with or without subsequent radiotherapy, to formal clearance. The combination of a complete axillary clearance with radiotherapy causes unacceptable arm oedema and is now avoided.

The major lymphatic drainage of the breast is to the axilla and the axillary nodes are divided into three levels (Fig. 1.5).

There are, on average, 13.5 lymph nodes present at level I, 4.5 nodes at level II and 2.3 nodes at level III. Very few patients have lymph nodes involved at level II or level III in the absence of level I involvement. These so-called skip metastases occurred in only 1.3% of patients who were axillary node positive in a large series published from Milan.

Axillary node status remains the single best prognostic factor and important treatment decisions are based upon it. In addition the axilla needs treatment to prevent uncontrolled local disease. This can be provided either by surgery or radiotherapy, although using the latter without knowing if the nodes contain tumour means that some people will receive radiotherapy unnecessarily.

How much surgery and for whom is also controversial. Clinical examination of the axilla correlates badly with true nodal status as assessed histologically; some form of sampling is therefore needed. There are, as yet, no good imaging techniques for the axilla and this is one area where a major advance is needed. (Early reports on the use of magnetic resonance imaging sound promising.)

Role of axillary surgery

The role of axillary surgery is twofold:

● To stage the axilla
● To treat axillary disease

Other techniques of staging the axilla including clinical examination and various radiological techniques are unsatisfactory. Surgical options which have been described in the axilla include: a single-node biopsy; an axillary node sample — removing four nodes from the axilla; axillary dissection to a landmark such as the intercostobrachial nerve; a level I dissection; a level II dissection; and a level III dissection.

Staging of the axilla is also important for selection of adjuvant therapy, providing prognostic information and providing an index of efficacy of screening programmes.

Ability of these procedures to stage the axilla

It is clear that a single node biopsy does not adequately stage the axilla. Similarly axillary dissection to a particular landmark, (the one which has been most commonly used being the intercostobrachial nerve), is also inaccurate in assessing whether the patient is node positive. Much debate has surrounded the use of axillary node sampling. Data from Edinburgh on 401 patients undergoing a mastectomy and randomized to either an axillary node sample or an axillary node clearance showed that the axillary node sample group had a node positivity rate of 42% whereas those undergoing clearance had a node positivity rate of 40%. This suggests that both are equally effective at staging the axilla. This is supported by further data on 135 patients who having undergone an axillary node sample were then randomized to have either a clearance or no more surgery. Of the 67 patients who initially underwent sampling and then went on to have a clearance, 41 patients were node negative on the sample; none of these converted to node positive on the clearance.

Using data from Milan a mathematical model has been formulated to determine the number of nodes which have to be present in a level I sample to have a 90% chance of predicting true node-negative status. This mathematical model suggests that at least 10 nodes have to be

Table 6.6   Correlation of number of involved axillary nodes at level I with percentage of patients who will have involved nodes at levels II and III

Number positive at level I	% with positive nodes at level II and III
1	12
2	19
3	37
4	40
5	84

sampled. The problem with these data and results from other similar studies are that they presume that all nodes in the axilla are equally likely to be sampled. Data from this mathematical model indicate that when only five nodes are sampled at level I then there would only be a 73% chance of picking up all node-positive patients. If this model were applied to the data from the Edinburgh randomized study, 10 out of 41 patients classified as node negative should have had unrecognized positive nodes. None actually did. This model also predicts that four-node sampling should not be a satisfactory procedure in staging the axilla, and yet clinical data clearly indicate it is. In node sampling it is the four largest nodes which are sampled which differs from a level I dissection where all axillary fat and lymph nodes are removed within the anatomical boundaries of level I (Fig. 1.5). The mathematical model probably does apply if a formal anatomical level I dissection is performed, in which case a minimum of 10 nodes are needed to be certain that the axillary disease is accurately staged. Axillary dissection to level II or level III is effective at assessing the axillary lymph node status as the majority or all nodes are removed from the axilla. An axillary node sample (4 nodes), a level I dissection (10 nodes) or a level II and III clearance will all adequately stage the axilla.

Treatment of axillary disease
There are two main options for treating the involved axilla:

- Radical radiotherapy
- Full level III axillary clearance

Even in patients with one node positive at level I, there is a significant chance of nodes at level II or III being involved (Table 6.6); and this chance increases as the number of positive nodes at level I increases. A level I dissection alone can, therefore, never be considered a therapeutic procedure in a patient who has even a single axillary nodal metastasis. The same problem arises with a level II dissection in that 50% of those with level II

Table 6.7   Control of axillary disease from National Surgical Adjuvant Breast Project Protocol B-O4

	Clinically node +ve		Clinically node −ve	
	Mx Cl	Mx XRT	Mx Cl	Mx XRT
% axillary recurrence	1	11.9	1.4	3.1

Mx = mastectomy, Cl = axillary node clearance, XRT = radiotherapy

Table 6.8   Morbidity after axillary procedures

	XRT	Cl	NS
Lymphoedema	+	+	0
Nerve problems	+	+	0/ +
Sarcomas	+	0	0
ROM at shoulder	+ / + +	+	0/ +

XRT = radiotherapy, Cl = axillary clearance, NS = axillary node sample, ROM = range of movement

involvement also have disease at level III. A level II dissection thus gives no more information than can be gleaned from an axillary node sample or a level I dissection and does not adequately treat the involved axilla.

Studies of axillary recurrence generally indicate that in patients with involved axillary nodes, axillary clearance provides lower recurrence rates than radical radiotherapy (Table 6.7). These differences are, however, not dramatic and a 95% control rate of disease in the axilla at 8 years in patients with involved nodes is possible using radiotherapy.

Morbidity of radiotherapy and axillary clearance

The complications include lymphoedema and damage to nerves in the axilla (surgically this is division of the intercostobrachial, long thoracic or thoracodorsal nerves and with radiotherapy there is the rare complication of brachial plexothapy). Another problem with radiotherapy is that it can induce sarcomas. Both surgery and radiotherapy also have effects in reducing the range of movement of the shoulder. The incidence of these complications is summarized in Table 6.8. The aim in the axilla must be to limit morbidity as well as achieve disease control.

There are some who believe that surgeons should not enter the axilla. This group suggests that clinically involved axillae should be treated with radical radiotherapy and in the remainder a watch policy should be adopted, treating only those patients who develop symptomatic axillary relapse. Administering radiotherapy to the axillae of all patients with palpable axillary nodes ignores the fact that up to 40% will not have axillary node involvement and will thus be receiving unnecessary treatment which is associated with significant morbidity. Important information in deciding adjuvant treatment and prognosis is also not obtained.

The watch policy, treating disease only when it becomes clinically evident is based on the findings of the NSABP B-O4, which randomized patients who were clinically axillary node negative to receive a mastectomy and axillary node clearance, mastectomy and radiotherapy, or a mastectomy alone. The results of this study are summarized in the Table 6.9. As can be seen, only 18% of those who did not have either full axillary clearance or radiotherapy subsequently developed axillary relapse, and there were no differences between the groups in overall survival at 10 years. There are, however, a number of problems with this study in that one-third of the mastectomy group who apparently received mastectomy alone did have a limited axillary dissection. Although over 20% of patients developed symptomatic axillary disease if no nodes were excised during the mastectomy, this was reduced to 8% if there was a very limited lower axillary dissection whereas no one had symptomatic disease if more than five nodes were removed as part of the mastectomy. It was also evident that a number of patients in the mastectomy-only group who developed axillary recurrence had uncontrollable axillary disease.

Predicting which patients will have involved axillary nodes

There is a direct relationship between tumour size and the presence of lymph node metastases (Fig. 5.5). It is of interest that tumours detected by screening are less likely to have axillary metastases at each individual size than symptomatic patients. For this reason it has become standard practice in many units for patients with impalpable breast cancer to perform an axillary node sample or a level I dissection, whereas those with palpable disease are treated with a level III clearance. For patients undergoing a mastectomy for invasive breast cancer an axillary clearance is indicated, thus reducing the need for postoperative radiotherapy in the majority. This is particularly important when immediate breast reconstruction is being performed as radiotherapy will significantly affect the final cosmetic result. This goes someway to meeting the aims of limiting the morbidity of surgery and/or radiotherapy to those who require it. It is evident that if the patient is node negative then it would be best to identify this group by the most limited surgery, such as an axillary node sample, whereas in patients who are node positive it would be ideal for them to have an axillary node clearance as this would both stage and treat the axilla. What is required are preoperative assessments which will allow those patients with axillary node disease to be identified. At present no such investigations are available.

Table 6.9 Axillary recurrence following clearance, radiotherapy and watch policy (from National Surgical Adjuvant Breast Protocol B-04)

	Mx Cl	Mx XRT	Mx
Number of patients	362	352	365
% axillary relapse	1	3	18
10-year survival	46	48	41

Mx = mastectomy, Cl = axillary node clearance, XRT = radiotherapy

Techniques of axillary surgery

Axillary node sampling. This is usually performed through a separate axillary incision in the skin crease of the axilla and should ideally be undertaken immediately prior to the wide local excision. The axilla is entered and the tail of the breast and lower axilla palpated. If nodes cannot be identified easily, the edges of pectoralis major and latissimus dorsi muscles should be formally identified and a finger passed round behind the lower axillary fat, which is situated between these two muscles; this makes nodes in this fat easier to feel. Starting from the lower axilla at least four palpable nodes are excised and sent separately for histology. If four nodes are not palpable in the lower axilla (level I) then palpable nodes from higher in the axilla (level II, level III or the interpectoral region, see Fig. 1.5) are excised. It is important to appreciate that an axillary node sample is not merely a level I dissection but samples palpable nodes from any level of the axilla. This should allow detection of the few patients who have level II or III involvement but uninvolved level I axillary nodes, the so-called skip metastases. Haemostasis in the axilla is secured with diathermy. No drains are necessary and the wound is closed in layers with absorbable sutures.

Axillary node clearance. Prior to the start of the operation the arm is draped so it can be moved during the procedure. As with axillary node sampling, axillary node clearance is usually performed through a separate incision, before the wide local excision. A lazy S incision is made along the skin creases of the axilla. The skin incision is deepened and skin flaps dissected to the edges of the pectoralis major and latissimus dorsi muscles. The pectoralis minor muscle is cleared of tissue. This is best performed with the arm placed above the patient's head with retraction on the pectoralis major muscle if the pectoralis minor muscle is not to be divided. If there is evidence of extensive nodal disease, division of pectoralis minor on the coracoid process allows a more thorough clearance to be performed. The front of the axillary vein is identified and the contents of the axilla below the vein are cleared to the apex of the axilla preserving the long thoracic nerve, the thoracodorsal nerve and vessels and, if possible, the intercostobrachial nerve. A combination of blunt and sharp dissection, with division of structures between ligaclips, allows a speedy and effective clearance of the axilla. The undersurface of the pectoralis major muscle should be carefully palpated and any palpable interpectoral nodes excised. Dissection of the lower axillary contents should continue into the axillary tail of the breast. A single suction drain is placed in the axilla and remains in situ until the volume of fluid in the drain is less than 50 ml in 24 h. The wound is closed with absorbable sutures.

ADJUVANT SYSTEMIC TREATMENT

This is aimed at the second fundamental part of breast cancer treatment (attempting to reduce the systemic load) and requires the administration of an intervention (chemotherapy, endocrine therapy or endocrine ablation) to an otherwise well patient. These treatments all have potential side-effects and a risk-benefit analysis needs making on the patient's behalf.

The translation of benefits for such treatments from large trials which have shown improvements in overall survival and time to relapse to an individual can be difficult for both patient and clinician. A node-positive woman who relapses at, for example, 36 months despite receiving adjuvant chemotherapy may not feel that 6 months of chemotherapy was worthwhile even if, statistically, she would otherwise have relapsed at 24 months.

The role of chemotherapy and endocrine therapy is now reasonably well established and newer agents are being studied. The arguments that raged 5 years ago, between those who felt there was a benefit for patients receiving adjuvant chemotherapy and those who believed that the results were unimpressive and the toxicity high, have largely disappeared with the publication of large well-controlled trials. Although individually these pointed to the benefits for chemotherapy, only when pooled as an overview was the actual level of benefit for both chemotherapy and tamoxifen apparent. This overview published in the Lancet in early 1992 is discussed further in the chapter 9.

Adjuvant chemotherapy

Combination chemotherapy (such as cyclophosphamide, methotrexate and 5-fluorouracil; CMF) reduces the odds of early recurrence and death. This is most marked for premenopausal, node-positive patients where a 25% reduction in the odds of dying before 10 years is achievable. The benefit translates into a prolongation of life (probably of the

Table 6.10   Common adjuvant chemotherapy regimens

Regimen	Dose
*CMF** repeated every 28 days	
cyclophosphamide	100 mg/m^2 orally days 1–14 or 500 mg/m^2 intravenously days 1 and 8
methotrexate	35 mg/m^2 intravenously days 1 and 8
5-fluorouracil	600 mg/m^2 intravenously days 1 and 8
An alternative regimen repeated every 21 days is:	
cyclophosphamide	600 mg/m^2 intravenously day 1 only
methotrexate	35 mg/m^2 intravenously day 1
5-fluorouracil	600 mg/m^2 intravenously day 1
MMM repeated every 21 days	
methotrexate	40 mg/m^2 intravenously
mitozantrone	7 mg/m^2 intravenously
mitomycin-C	7 mg/m^2 intravenously
FAC repeated every 21 days	
5-fluorouracil	600 mg/m^2 intravenously
adriamycin	60 mg/m^2 intravenously
cyclophosphamide	600 mg/m^2 intravenously
FEC substitutes epirubicin for adriamycin at a dose of 60 mg/m^2	
Single agent epirubicin	
epirubicin	20 mg intravenously every 7 or 14 days

* There are many variations on CMF regimes

order of 2–3 years) for 25% of the 40% who would not have been cured by surgery and radiotherapy alone, i.e. about a 10% absolute increase in survival. For node-negative premenopausal ladies the benefit is less clear (hence the attempts to use prognostic factors as decision making tools). In postmenopausal ladies tamoxifen is the most widely used form of adjuvant treatment and achieves similar levels of benefit to that of chemotherapy in premenopausal women. There may still be a place for chemotherapy in the node-positive postmenopausal group of women.

Combination chemotherapy is more effective than single agent regimens and are traditionally given for six cycles. Some of the commonly used regimens are shown in Table 6.10. The jury is still out on the question of whether improvements in survival can be obtained by increasing the dose of drug administered (dose intensification), but it does appear that four cycles of a 5-fluorouracil, adriamycin and cyclophosphamide (FAC) treatment, substituting the more active agent adriamycin (doxorubicin) for methotrexate, given at a higher dose is more effective than six cycles at a lower dose or six cycles of CMF. Further evidence for an improvement in survival with dose intensification is becoming available from the early results of the bone marrow transplantation programmes currently underway in America.

The drugs need to be given in a well-supervised unit by appropriately trained staff with protocols for the management of complications. There is no place for a pre-registration Houseman being left alone to give potentially dangerous drugs.

Complications of chemotherapy

The complications and side-effects include alopecia, neutropenia, nausea and vomiting. There are also specific side-effects for each agent which are not discussed here.

Alopecia. This can be expected with higher doses of cyclophosphamide and mitozantrone and at most commonly used doses of doxorubicin (adriamycin). This may be reduced by scalp cooling using either cold packs or, preferably, a purpose-built scalp cooling machine.

Neutropenia. This is to be expected and regular blood count should be obtained. The nadir (lowest point) for most regimens is known and patients may need prophylactic antibiotics to cover this period. Dose reductions and delays may be necessary if the white cell count falls below defined limits. The death of a patient through uncontrolled infection due to neutropenia offsets any benefit in reduction of mortality for the population being treated. The use of haematological growth factors prepared by genetic engineering techniques can shorten the time a patient is neutropenic and reduce the need for antibiotics. Granulocyte colony stimulating factor (G-CSF) is more commonly used than GM-CSF (macrophages included) but the exact role of these growth factors is currently being evaluated.

Nausea and vomiting. These are among the more unpleasant side-effects of chemotherapy. The percentage of patients experiencing nausea differs with the different combinations of chemotherapy and some regimens require few or no antiemetic measures. Others, such as cisplatin, Dacarbazine and high-dose doxorubicin are highly emetogenic. Recognized antiemetic regimens are shown in Table 6.11. The arrival of the 5-HT$_3$ receptor antagonists has (at a cost) reduced the problem to manageable levels. It seems reasonable to reserve these agents for highly emetogenic regimens and for those whose nausea cannot be controlled by more conventional measures such as sea-bands (which use stimulation of the P5 acupuncture point on the volar aspect of the wrist), regular metoclopramide, benzodiazapines, dexamethasone, and cannabis derivatives.

Younger women are more at risk of nausea and vomiting. The aim of treatment is to prevent them ever experiencing it so as to avoid the condition of anticipatory nausea and vomiting which can be particularly upsetting.

Table 6.11   Antiemetic regimes for chemotherapy-induced nausea and vomiting

Regimen	Administration
Low emetogenic regimes (low-dose epirubicin)	Oral metoclopramide (if necessary)
Moderately emetogenic regimens (CMF, MMM doxorubicin, high-dose epirubicin)	Dexamethasone 8–16 mg intravenously before or after chemotherapy and metoclopramide* followed by oral dexamethasone (4 mg t.d.s. for 3 days) and metoclopramide (10 mg t.d.s. for 3 days) to take at home. Metoclopramide may be continued if necessary. If this fails then ondansetron 8 mg intravenously or granisetron 3 mg intravenously before chemotherapy with dexamethasone intravenously and followed by oral dexamethasone.
Highly emetogenic regimens (not often used in routine management of breast cancer other than some centres using cisplatin regimens but used for high-dose doxorubicin and patients who fail on the above regimens)	Ondansetron 8 mg intravenously or granisetron 3 mg intravenously before chemotherapy with dexamethasone intravenously and followed by oral dexamethasone.

* low dose 20–30 mg intravenously or high dose 100 mg infusion — may need to give 1 mg benztropine intravenously in younger patients receiving high dose to combat extrapyramidal side-effects

Endocrine therapy

That oestrogens are involved in the processes of breast cancer induction, growth and metastasis is very clear. Measures that might reduce the levels or block the actions of oestrogen should, therefore, be beneficial. For premenopausal women removal of the ovaries (oophorectomy) is an effective way of reducing circulating oestrogens. This may be achieved by surgical removal or by radiotherapy (they are very radiosensitive). The ovaries can also be suppressed by the use of luteinizing hormone releasing hormone (LHRH) superagonists. These latter agents suppress ovarian secretion which lasts a day or two and the circulating level of oestrogen falls in the majority of women to the postmenopausal levels. Drugs in this category include goserelin (Zoladex, Zeneca; ICI) and leuprorelin (Prostap; Lederle).

In premenopausal women the overview data show that ovarian ablation confers the same order of reduction in the odds of death as chemotherapy. As amenorrhoea is one of the side-effects of chemotherapy, it has been suggested that part of its effect is through ovarian suppression. There are several trials ongoing to try and settle this issue.

The best known endocrine therapy is the 'anti-oestrogen' tamoxifen.

Developed by ICI as a possible contraceptive it was found to be both weakly oestrogenic and an anti-oestrogen in different tissues. It was used initially in the treatment of advanced breast cancer and found to be effective. It is thought to exert its action by disrupting the expression of the message generated when oestrogen binds to its receptor.

The Nolvadex Adjuvant Tamoxifen Organization (NATO) trial which randomized node-positive patients over the age of 50 to either 2 years of tamoxifen or no tamoxifen continues to show a survival benefit for those on tamoxifen. The CRC has repeated this study with 2230 stage I and II patients. Unlike the NATO study it included premenopausal and node-negative patients. It too demonstrated a major benefit (about 27% reduction in odds of relapse) for the tamoxifen treated group irrespective of tumour size, nodal status or age. How long tamoxifen needs to be given after surgery is currently being investigated. The original studies used 2 years but the overview has suggested that more may be better. Tamoxifen is well tolerated by patients and its side-effect profile is low although the anti-oestrogenic hot flushes and vaginal dryness can be a problem. This may be more of a problem for the premenopausal group which is increasingly being prescribed it. The vaginal dryness can be treated with a variety of medications including: local non-steroidal creams (K-Y jelly and Replens), local oestrogen creams and stopping the tamoxifen.

The high-risk patient

By definition, some individuals are at very high risk of early relapse and protocols of aggressive treatment for this group are being assessed. In the USA this includes studies of women with 10 or more positive nodes, some of whom are being offered high-dose chemotherapy with autologous bone marrow transplantation (ABMT) or peripheral stem cell harvesting. The early results show that treatment mortality is controllable (around 5%) although morbidity is high. There has been some prolongation of time to relapse but this has yet to translate into a survival benefit. This approach has yet to be widely taken up in the UK although ABMT is being offered to some ladies on relapse.

Use of adjuvant treatment

A suggestion of how patients might pragmatically be divided into groups for adjuvant treatment is shown in Table 6.12. This represents standard best treatment and may well change as further studies are reported. Paradoxically many centres actively involved in the treatment of patients with breast cancer may not use such a scheme as they may well be involved in clinical trials.

Table 6.12 Adjuvant therapy for patients with breast cancer

Menopausal and nodal status	Therapy
Premenopausal node negative	Nothing or tamoxifen (if high risk consider chemotherapy and/or ovarian manipulation)
Premenopausal node positive	Adjuvant chemotherapy
	< 4 nodes; CMF × 6 cycles
	4–10 nodes; FAC × 4 or × 6 cycles
	> 10 nodes; ?FAC, ?more intensive treatment
	Plus consider ovarian manipulation
Postmenopausal node negative	Most get tamoxifen
Postmenopausal node positive	Tamoxifen
	Consider chemotherapy if aggressive disease

TREATMENT OF BREAST CANCER DURING PREGNANCY

In these patients there can be a delay in making a diagnosis due to the difficulty of identifying a discrete mass within enlarging breasts. Bone scans should not be performed to stage the disease. A modified radical mastectomy is the standard treatment and radiotherapy is contraindicated during any trimester. Chemotherapy can been given during pregnancy but is associated with a small risk of fetal damage. During the third trimester treatment can be delayed until delivery of the baby (which is induced at 30–32 weeks), providing regular monitoring (ideally by ultrasound) shows no significant increase in size. Prognosis is similar stage for stage to women of the same age with breast cancer who are not pregnant.

TREATMENT OF PAGET'S DISEASE

In approximately 50% of patients Paget's disease is associated with a mass lesion (of which over 90% will turn out to be invasive ductal carcinoma). These should be treated by standard therapies such as a wide excision (including the nipple) with radiotherapy or mastectomy.

If there is no associated lump approximately 30% will have an invasive carcinoma at resection, the remainder having only DCIS or no detectable malignancy within the breast. Less than 10% of patients without a clinical mass will have nodal metastases whereas over 60% of those with a mass have axillary disease.

Care must be taken to distinguish between Paget's disease and direct spread of an invasive carcinoma to the skin of the nipple (Fig. 3.3B). Not only do they have different histological appearances but the treatment and outcome also differ. Pagets's disease may occupy a large area of the breast (Fig. 6.8).

Wide local excision for Paget's disease without a clinical or mammographic lesion has been proposed but is associated with a high incidence of recurrence which is often invasive. Whether wide excision and radiotherapy produces better local control is unclear. The recommended treatment for Paget's disease without a mass lesion is, therefore, a mastectomy and axillary node sample.

FOLLOW-UP OF BREAST CANCER PATIENTS

After treatment breast cancer patients are traditionally followed up at regular intervals. In the trial setting this is usually 3-monthly for the first 2 years, 6-monthly for the next 2 years and yearly thereafter. Some discharge patients from annual follow-up at 7 years, others at 10 years and some keep their patients returning until death or retirement arrives. This is somewhat illogical as recurrences are uncommon before 2 years. In addition, the majority of recurrences are detected by the patient between visits and not by the staff at the follow-up clinic. It is difficult to change this as patients themselves often like the reassurance of a visit where no disease is found. It is also pleasant to see some patients doing well; if all the successes are discharged one is left with only those who have recurrent disease which can make for a depressing clinic.

Routine follow-up consists of examination of the breast(s), axillae and supraclavicular fossa with palpation of the abdomen to elicit any hepatomegaly. Mammograms are usually performed 1 year after surgery and then either annually or every 2 years depending on type of disease and treatment. A reasonable protocol for follow-up is 6-monthly for 2 years and annually thereafter.

OTHER RARE NEOPLASMS

Lymphomas and sarcomas (malignant phyllodes tumours (cystosarcoma), fibrosarcoma and malignant fibrous histiocytoma, angiosarcoma, leiomyosarcoma, liposarcoma and osteosarcoma) occur in the breast but are rare. Sarcomas may develop in an area of breast or skin following radiotherapy. The diagnosis is often suggested by fine needle aspiration cytology. Lymphomas are treated by wide excision, radiotherapy and chemotherapy. Sarcomas are best widely excised by mastectomy and followed by radiotherapy, but there is no evidence that chemotherapy is of benefit.

Rare lesions which when excised recur locally include fibromatosis and nodular fasciitis. These have minimal malignant potential and are treated by wide excision.

7. Advanced disease

INTRODUCTION

Advanced disease is usually subdivided into locally advanced (i.e. locally inoperable) and metastatic. Metastatic breast cancer is incurable, although long-term and worthwhile short-term responses can be achieved by the use of appropriate treatment. It is important that quality of life is addressed in treating patients with advanced disease. Tools for measuring this are available and are used in research but have yet to find a place in the routine management of patients.

LOCALLY ADVANCED DISEASE

Definition

There are two groups of patients with locally advanced disease. The 'advanced by neglect' group whereby a slowly growing tumour has been ignored and allowed to become locally fixed or ulcerated. The other group is the true advanced disease and presents with fixed axillary nodes (N_2) or local signs such as peau d'orange (literally the skin of the orange) (Fig. 7.1) or the changes of an inflammatory carcinoma. Some include large T_3 tumours as advanced disease, which is inappropriate as many of these patients will have no evidence of disease elsewhere and can be adequately treated by mastectomy and radiotherapy. It is worthwhile staging this group of patients with bone and liver scans in addition to a chest X-ray (Table 6.3). If the disease is localized then surgery and/or radiotherapy may still be curative.

Increasingly primary systemic therapy is being offered. The aim is to downstage locally advanced disease. This may be achieved with tamoxifen if the patient is elderley or unfit, and a needle aspirate from the tumour has shown it to contain oestrogen receptors (ERs), or by (neoadjuvant) chemotherapy. Combination or high-dose single-agent doxorubicin chemotherapy has been shown to have a response rate of 80–90% and patients who respond may then be treated with either

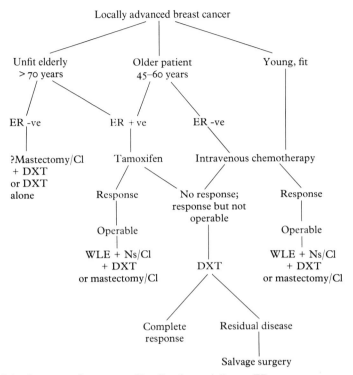

Fig. 7.2 Summary of treatment of locally advanced disease. ER = oestrogen receptor; WLE = wide local excision; Ns = axillary node sample; Cl = axillary node clearance; DXT = radiotherapy.

lumpectomy, quadrantectomy or mastectomy. The chemotherapy is usually given intravenously either as a bolus or by constant infusion; but it can also be given into the arteries feeding the breast — the internal mammary and lateral thoracic vessels. This latter technique results in high response rates which may be achievable in two cycles instead of the four needed for the intravenous route. As chemotherapy depends on an intact blood supply it seems logical to use it as an initial treatment followed by surgery if a good response is obtained. If the patient fails to respond to systemic or regional chemotherapy, or if the signs of local advancement are still present, then radiotherapy is an appropriate second treatment with surgery being used thereafter to remove any residual disease (salvage surgery). Figure 7.2 shows a summary of the options for the treatment of advanced breast cancer.

Table 7.1   Treatment of local recurrence

Type of recurrence	Treatment
Single spot	Excise
	consider radiotherapy
Multiple spot	More radical excision + / − flap
	radiotherapy if none previously
Widespread recurrence	Restage
	Intra-arterial chemotherapy
	Systemic therapy
	hormone therapy
	chemotherapy (?infusional 5-fluorouracil)

Histological examination of specimens resected after induction chemotherapy often show viable tumour cells even if a complete response has been seen clinically. Failure to follow a clinically complete response to chemotherapy with other local treatments results in high rates of local relapse.

LOCALLY RECURRENT DISEASE

The treatment of local recurrences after conservation surgery is discussed on page 112. Recurrence after mastectomy usually occurs in the skin flaps adjacent to the scar and is presumed to arise from viable cells shed at the time of surgery. If radiotherapy was not given at the time of mastectomy it can be used after excision of the recurrence. If the recurrence is small and occurs many years after the original surgery, excision alone may provide control. If the recurrence is in a previously irradiated field more extensive surgery should be entertained as further radiotherapy will often not be possible (Table 7.1). Standard chemo-therapy in this situation is disappointing presumably because the blood supply is diminished although the intra-arterial route may give higher concentrations. 5-fluorouracil infused continuously into a central vein via a Hickman line appears to be effective in local recurrence which has proved resistant to more standard treatments. Radical surgery may require resection of underlying structures and reconstruction with flaps. Failure to achieve local control may lead to cancer-en-cuirasse where the chest wall is encircled by tumour — a most unpleasant situation for the patient as the tumour often smells or bleeds. Local recurrence can be quite indolent, growing slowly without obvious metastasis elsewhere.

Recurrence in the axilla (usually termed loco-regional relapse) can be treated by surgical clearance if this has not been performed but is associated with the risk of postoperative lymphoedema. If the nodes are fixed it may be impossible to operate safely and radiotherapy may be more appropriate if it has not already been given.

Recurrence in the supraclavicular nodes represents dissemination but can often be controlled by radiotherapy. Local surgery has little to contribute in this situation except in making the diagnosis which may be more expeditiously achieved by needle cytology.

Systemic therapy has a role in the treatment of local relapse and should be considered if staging investigations show evidence of dissemination. Local disease may respond if the tumour remains chemosensitive.

METASTATIC DISEASE

Metastatic disease may present initially with local recurrence or as dissemination alone.

Whilst some patients have metastatic disease at the time of presentation, the majority have previously been diagnosed and treated. The median time to relapse for aggressive disease is around 2 years. The site of relapse is important as tumours which relapse in bone and soft tissue respond better to treatment than those relapsing in liver, brain or lung. A recurrence in the original surgical field may not always be accompanied by metastatic spread and, if staging tests are negative, it can be dealt with by resection and radiotherapy (Table 7.1).

If surgical control of local recurrence cannot be achieved, or if widespread metastatic disease is present, then alternative treatments are needed. If the disease is advancing rapidly and is life threatening (for instance if there are liver and/or lung metastases) then combination chemotherapy is indicated. If not, then endocrine treatments should be tried first. Some idea of how likely a response will be can be gleaned from the disease free interval (DFI). Patients with a short DFI are less likely to respond to hormonal therapy.

The original endocrine treatment was oophorectomy (described for the treatment of advanced breast cancer by Beatson in 1896) and was followed by the apparant paradoxical use of the synthetic oestrogen, diethyl stilboestrol, in the 1940s. This proved effective but was associated with high rates of thromboembolic phenomena. Both adrenalectomy and hypophysectomy were found to be effective treatments in animals and were used in humans in the 1950s. Their use has been superseded by the anti-oestrogen tamoxifen and the aromatase inhibitors aminoglutethimide and 4-hydroxyandrostenedione (4OHA). These latter compounds block the conversion of androgens to oestrogen. Aminoglutethimide is less specific in its action, working earlier in the conversion process and, although initially it was given in combination with hydrocortisone to prevent a reflex rise in adrenocorticotrophic hormone secretion, it is now used in lower doses without hydrocortisone. It has a much higher rate of side-effects when compared with tamoxifen, the most common being a skin rash occurring between 10–14 days. The newer agent 4OHA can only be given by injection although other forms are being developed. A pure anti-oestrogen has also been developed and is undergoing trials. Other oral endocrine agents include medroxyprogesterone acetate (MPA), megestrol and steroids.

The luteinizing hormone releasing hormone (LHRH) superagonists goserelin and leuprorelin have also been used in patients with advanced disease with response rates in the order of 30%.

Endocrine therapy in metastatic disease is most likely to be effective if there has been a long DFI and if the original tumour was ER positive. The options for patients are as follows:

- Premenopausal
  Oophorectomy
  Surgical or radiation induced.
  LHRH agonist
  Goserlin 3.6 mg monthly subcutaneously.
  Leuprorelin 3.75 mg monthly subcutaneously or intramuscularly.
- Postmenopausal
  No previous tamoxifen
  Tamoxifen 20 mg orally once a day.
  Previous tamoxifen
  Megestrol 160 mg orally once a day.
  Medroxyprogesterone acetate 1000 mg orally once a day or 500–1000 mg intramuscularly daily.
  Aminoglutethimide 1000 mg plus 40 mg hydrocortisone orally or 250–500 mg with no hydrocortisone.
  4OHA 250 mg intramuscularly every 2 weeks.

Response rates (complete and partial) are in the region of 30–40%. In patients who have responded to one endocrine agent but subsequently relapse, a second hormonal agent should be tried as long as the disease has not become life threatening. Prednisolone 40 mg/day may be tried in addition to, or instead of, the above agents but should be discontinued unless a response is seen in 2 weeks.

Combination chemotherapy is given in a similar manner to adjuvant therapy although different agents may be used. Again aggressive disease needs treating aggressively with an anthracycline containing regimen (doxorubicin or epirubicin, e.g. FAC or FEC) with the triple M (MMM — mitomycin C, methotrexate and mitozantrone) being an option if the patient has already had CMF as adjuvant treatment. Response rates of around 30% may be seen although this can be increased with dose escalation.

Novel ways of administering some of these agents are currently being developed. Continuous infusion of 5-fluorouracil over several months

Table 7.2 Treatment of metastatic breast cancer

Site of cancer	Treatment
Non-life threatening sites (bone, soft tissue)	Consider hormone manipulation initially Local radiotherapy for pain May need chemotherapy if short disease-free interval, ER negative or obviously symptomatic
Life threatening sites	
Liver, lung	Systemic chemotherapy (CMF, MMM, FAC etc.) If young, dose intensification (bone marrow transplantation or peripheral stem cell harvesting for rescue) If elderly, low-dose epirubicin, oral anthracycline or tamoxifen if not already tried
Brain	Steroids plus consider radiotherapy Excision if isolated metastasis

using a small pump and a Hickman line has shown promising results. This is well tolerated apart from the side-effect of the hand–foot syndrome where an erythematous rash is seen.

Bone marrow transplantation after high-dose chemotherapy is being evaluated in selected young patients with metastatic breast cancer and does seem to offer higher response rates and longer time to relapse.

Older and less fit patients may be treated by weekly or fortnightly epirubicin at 20 mg/m^2. A newer orally ingestible anthracycline is available on the Continent and may be useful for this group. Care has to be taken in monitoring side-effects as the elderly are less tolerent of a neutropenia. The treatment of metastatic breast cancer is summarized in Table 7.2.

TREATMENT OF THE ELDERLY OR UNFIT

Fit elderly patients should be treated in an identical manner to younger women. If the patient is reluctant or unfit for surgery tamoxifen treatment can be given as primary therapy. Trials of tamoxifen versus surgery for the elderly have shown that although some tumours respond well to tamoxifen alone, with complete and long-term partial responses, the majority eventually relapse on this treatment and need resection or radiotherapy. Some units would only consider giving tamoxifen to patients whose tumours contain high levels of ER as this is the group most likely to respond. This can be determined on fine needle aspiration cytology samples using an ER immunocytochemical assay. In centres where this is not available an empirical course of tamoxifen is often tried with a change of management if no response is seen. If a tumour

Table 7.3 Performance status. Karnofsky and WHO grading

	WHO criteria		Karnofsky
0	Able to carry on normal activity	100	Normal; no complaints; no evidence of disease
		90	Able to carry on normal activity; minor signs of disease
1	Patient able to live at home with tolerable tumour manifestation	80	Normal activity with effort; some signs and symptoms of disease
		70	Cares for self; unable to carry on normal activity
2	Patient with disabling tumour manifestations but < 50% of time in bed	60	Requires occasional assistance but can care for most of her needs
		50	Requires considerable assistance and much medical care
3	Patient severely disabled and > 50% of time in bed but able to stand up	40	Disabled; requires special care
		30	Severely disabled; hospitilization but death not imminent
4	Patient very sick and bedridden	20	Very sick; active support and hospital treatment needed
		10	Moribund, fatal processes progressing rapidly
5	Dead	5	Dead

has responded to tamoxifen and subsequently relapses the alternatives are either to try second-line endocrine therapy with agents such as Megace, medroxyprogesterone acetate, aminoglutethimide or the newer agent 4OHA and/or to surgery and radiotherapy.

Patients unfit for a general anaesthetic may be suitable for a local anaesthetic.

ASSESSMENT OF RESPONSE

The commonly used outcome measures include relapse-free and overall survival. These are usually well defined but should be used in conjunction with some assessment of quality of life. The performance status (a crude measure of how well the patient is) is usually quoted on the Karnofsky or World Health Organization (WHO) score and can be used to see if treatment improves physical symptoms (Table 7.3).

Toxicity of treatments are well quantified using the WHO grades (Table 7.4) and should be used to specify toxicity in trials or new treatments. The median duration of response of any treatment is when 50% of patients treated have relapsed and gives some idea of efficacy.

The response of a tumour is generally given in terms of a complete

Table 7.4 Simplified WHO grading system for toxicity of therapy

	Grade				
	0	1	2	3	4
Haemoglobin	> 11.0	9.5–11	8.0–9.4	6.5–7.9	< 6.5g/dl
Leucocytes	> 4.0	3.0–3.9	2.0–2.9	1.0–1.9	< 1x10⁹/L
Platelets	> 100	75–99	50–74	25–49	< 25x10⁹/L
Nausea/ vomiting	None	Nausea	Transient vomiting	Therapy needed	Intractable
Hair loss	No change	Minimal	Patchy alopecia	Complete alopecia	Irreversible

response (CR), partial response (PR), disease stabilization (DS) and disease progression (DP). There are well-defined criteria for each grouping based on International Union against Cancer (UICC) guidelines. These can be found in any oncology text. They are easier to apply when there is measurable disease such as a solitary metastasis but can be difficult to use if the disease is diffuse or if some areas are responding whilst others progress. With increasing use of primary systemic chemotherapy there is a need to assess the change of size of a tumour in the treated breast. This can be done with ultrasound and an estimate of tumour volume obtained from three-dimensional measurements.

Patients who respond to therapy do better and can achieve long-term control of their disease. Those who do not respond need alternative therapies but rarely do so well.

MALE BREAST CANCER

Male breast is over 100 times less common than the female variety and represents only 0.7% of all cancers which occur in men. One male breast cancer is seen for every 200 female breast cancers and thus represents 0.5% of all breast cancers. The peak age incidence is 5–10 years older than that in females. The aetiology, like that of female breast cancer, is unknown but there is an increased incidence in patients with Klinefelter syndrome. Gynaecomastia does not seem to be a risk factor.

Clinical features

The presenting features are identical to those in females, patients presenting with a lump, skin or nipple retraction and occasionally nipple discharge. The only difference between the sexes is that in male breast cancers infiltrate skin and the nipple early due to the smaller breast volume (Fig. 6.9).

The histology of male breast cancer is similar to that in the female and even invasive lobular carcinoma has been reported.

Prognosis

The outlook for male breast cancer is similar to that of the female when compared stage for stage but, as noted, the male tends to present with later stage disease.

Treatment

The preferred treatment is a modified radical mastectomy. Often this has to be followed by radiotherapy because of the narrower margins of excision and the often locally advanced nature of the disease. Although the hormonal milieu is different in males, breast cancer still appears to respond well to hormonal therapy and many tumours in males are ER positive. Tamoxifen is therefore the systemic adjuvant treatment of choice following excisional surgery and/or radiotherapy.

For metastatic breast cancer, the options include castration and chemotherapy.

SPECIFIC PROBLEMS SEEN IN PATIENTS WITH ADVANCED DISEASE

These include: hypercalcaemia; pathological fractures; pain; breathlessness from pleural or pulmonary disease; and raised intracranial pressure from cerebral secondaries.

Hypercalcaemia

This may be unrecognized but should be suspected in any patient with breast cancer who appears confused or complains of thirst and lassitude. Recent research has implicated a parathyroid hormone-related protein as the probable cause of the hypercalcaemia. Not all patients with advanced metastatic disease will develop it and some patients with apparently early disease may experience hypercalcaemia. Thirst, lassitude and confusion are, unfortunately, late symptoms and some of the 10–20% of women who develop hypercalcaemia during their illness go unrecognized. The majority of cases are associated with symptomatic bony metastases and a calcium level should be checked in such patients.

Many with hypercalcaemia are dehydrated and large volumes of saline may be needed to correct this. Saline is the most appropriate fluid for rehydration as sodium is linked to calcium excretion in the kidney and thus encourages renal disposal of some of the excess calcium. The addition of diuretics such as frusemide was recommended at one time, but is not now considered necessary. Restoration of normovolaemia usually results in a marked improvement in the patient's condition and the serum calcium may fall to normal levels. This will not provide lasting control and further measures are indicated. The use of the bisphosphonate compounds has significantly improved management of hypercalcaemia and have superseded agents such as steroids, phosphates and mithramycin which were previously used. The bisphoponates restore normocalcaemia in 2–3 days but may have to be repeated after a period varying from 2–3 weeks to 3 months to maintain this response unless the tumour concomitantly responds to therapy. They have to be given by intravenous infusion in the acute phase although maintenance therapy may be achieved by the oral route. The gut absorption is, however, poor and only one compound (clodrinate) is available for oral use.

Fractures

Bone is one of the most common sites of metastasis and will fracture if weakened sufficiently. Pathological fractures may need surgery to stabilize them and this may be an effective way of restoring pain-free mobility. If a metastasis is in a site that is likely to fracture, prophylactic pinning or other stabilization procedures may be useful. If a fracture is not in a site which will be helped by surgery then palliative radiotherapy is usually highly effective in relieving pain. This may be given either as a single fraction or as a short course to the painful area. Pain relief is often of good duration and quality which results in reduced needs for analgesics. Bisphosphonates appear to decrease pain and assist healing of pathological fractures.

The young woman who presents with symptomatic bony metastases can be treated with a LHRH agonist, oophorectomy or systemic chemotherapy. It is startling how effective an oophorectomy can be — the patient may wake up from the operation pain free (why this should be is unclear as the half-life of the circulating oestrogen is 17 h!). The response usually occurs in those patients who have a cancer with high ER levels and a trial of LHRH therapy should be instituted prior to oophorectomy.

Fractures or deposits in the spine may lead to spinal cord compression which is a true medical emergency as prompt diagnosis and treatment may prevent paraplegia. The most common presentation is for a patient to 'go off her legs' but pins and needles and an altered sensation are often found prior to this stage. Although magnetic resonance imaging is the best technique for assessing this group it is not yet freely available and most patients need a myelogram to determine the level of the block. Surgery to decompress the cord, with or without fixation by plating or grafting, and subsequent radiotherapy is the usual treatment along with a change in systemic therapy.

Cerebral metastases

These may cause distressing symptoms and are treated with dexamethasone (4 mg q.d.s.) to reduce the swelling (often responsible for the symptoms). Occasionally craniotomy to excise a solitary metastasis is indicated but recurrence is common. Cranial radiotherapy can delay recurrence of symptoms if a good response to dexamethasone is seen but is accompanied by side-effects of nausea and total alopecia. Even temporary restoration of normal faculties with these treatments is worthwhile, especially if this is the first sign of metastatic disease, as it may allow enough time for a patient to put their affairs in order.

SYMPTOM CONTROL AND PALLIATIVE CARE

Pain

60–70% of patients with advanced breast cancer complain of pain. Patients with metastatic cancer rarely have only one pain and the majority have several separate pains which may have different causes. Each site of pain should be identified and the underlying mechanism determined if possible. It is important to appreciate that the patient's emotional state (anger, despair, fear, anxiety, depression) may be important in how the patient responds to their pain. It is useful, therefore, to assess both the physical and emotional aspects of the patient's pain. Three stages of pain control have been described:

- to be pain free at night,
- to be pain free at rest, and
- to be pain free on movement.

While it is often possible to achieve the first two, the third may be difficult where there is widespread skeletal involvement. Analgesic approach to pain relief should be simple and flexible. Pain can be considered as mild, moderate and severe; appropriate treatments for these are outlined in Table 7.5.

Simple analgesics and opioids

Many patients do not receive an adequate trial of simple analgesics but, where they are ineffective, regular weak opioids such a co-proxamol or

Table 7.5 Choice of anlagesic for pain control

Pain severity	Class of analgesic	Preferred drug
Mild pain	Simple analgesic	Paracetemol (preferable to aspirin because of lack of gastrointestinal side-effects)
Moderate pain	Weak opioid analgesic (alone or in combination with simple analgesic)	Co-proxamol or codeine + paracetemol
Severe pain	Strong opioid analgesic	Morphine

dihydrocodeine should be the next therapeutic step before proceeding to a strong opioid.

Strong opioid analgesics

Morphine remains the strong opioid analgesic of choice for severe pain. Dose requirements vary widely from one patient to another but the dose should be started low and titrated against the pain until control is achieved. During dose titration aqueous morphine elixir should be used because it has a rapid onset and a short duration of action, but once stable dose requirements have been determined controlled release preparations, such as morphine (slow release) given twice or three times daily, are more convenient and improve patient compliance. An identical daily dose of slow release morphine (such as MST) should be substituted once the correct dose has been found. If breakthrough pain occurs during treatment with slow release preparations, morphine elixir can be added; although, if breakthrough pain is a frequent problem then the dose of MST should be increased.

It should be appreciated that slow release preparations should not be used for acute pain, as peak plasma concentrations of morphine are not reached for 2–4 h following administration. If medication cannot be given by mouth, rectal administration is an alternative route using the same dose and frequency as oral administration.

Parenteral opioids are not more effective than oral opioids although a smaller dose is required. The dose of oral morphine should be halved to give an equivalent dose of parenteral morphine. As diamorphine is more soluble than morphine the dose of oral morphine should be divided by three to obtain an equivalent dose for parenteral administration. Morphine can be delivered subcutaneously using a continuous infusion pump.

None of the other strong opioid analgesics have advantages which make them preferable to morphine.

Table 7.6 Adjuvant drugs in pain control

Cause of pain	Useful adjuvant drugs
Bone pain	NSAIDs, bisphosphonates
Soft tissue infiltration	NSAIDs or steroids
Hepatic enlargement	Steroids
Raised intracranial pressure	Steroids
Nerve compression or infiltration	Steroids
	Antidepressants
	Anticonvulsants
Muscle spasm	Diazepam
	Baclofen
Fungating tumour	Antibiotics (metronidazole)
Cellulitis	Antibiotics

NSAIDS = non-steroidal anti-inflammatory drugs

Side-effects of morphine

The common side-effects are drowsiness, constipation, nausea, vomiting and dry mouth. Drowsiness is usually only a problem at the start of treatment or when doses are increased; it usually resolves within a few days, when the dose has been stabilized. Constipation is a universal side-effect and all patients taking morphine should receive a regular laxative. Nausea and vomiting occur in a half to two-thirds of patients, and the preferable antiemetic is haloperidol given once or twice daily in a dose of 1.5 mg. Respiratory depression and addiction do not occur in cancer patients.

Adjuvant drugs

These may not have intrinsic analgesic activity but contribute significantly to pain relief when used in combination with a conventional analgesic (Table 7.6). Anxiety, depression, fear, restlessness and insomnia can all significantly reduce a patient's pain threshold and these symptoms often respond to benzodiazepine medication. Diazepam is the preferred oral anxiolytic, temazepam the hypnotic of choice and midazolam the choice for parenteral use. This latter drug which can be given by subcutaneous infusion is particularly useful in the management of terminal restlessness. The place of antidepressants in the management of chronic pain is not clear but some patients with advanced or terminal malignant disease do appear to respond to them.

Anticonvulsants are of value for lancinating or stabbing dysaesthetic pains associated with nerve infiltration or compression, postsurgical neuralgia, postherpetic neuralgia and other forms of neuropathic pain. Side-effects may be a problem with these drugs and so the initial dose should be low and titrated against the effects. The drug of choice is carbamazepine, initially starting at a dose of 100 mg twice a day and increasing to 800 mg per day.

Control of other symptoms

Lymphoedema. Upper limb lymphoedema is frequently encountered in patients with local recurrence in the axilla and supraclavicular regions. It may also occur as a complication of surgery or radiotherapy in the absence of local recurrence. It is a difficult problem to treat and often causes considerable pain and discomfort. In the first instance an elastic stocking or sleeve should be used in conjuction with other measures which include massage, limb exercise, compression bandaging and the use of intermittent compression sleeve devices.

Anorexia. Alcohol, corticosteroids and progestogens are the most helpful pharmacological treatments.

Dysphagia. This may occur because of oropharyngeal candidiasis or as a result of local tumour infiltration. The specific cause should therefore be sought. Treatment for candida includes nystatin suspension, amphotericin lozenges or fluconazole. External beam irradiation, surgical intubation or endoscopic laser therapy may be indicated where there is mechanical evidence of obstruction by tumour.

Nausea and vomiting. Nausea and vomiting may have many causes: drugs, uraemia, hepatic failure, hypercalcaemia, raised intercranial pressure and obstruction. Attention to the underlying cause and appropriate management with antiemetics is the mainstay of treatment.

Respiratory symptoms, lymphangitis carcinomatosa. Steroids are usually tried but are rarely effective. Non-specific symptomatic measures are the only option for the majority of patients.

Symptomatic treatment of dyspnoea. Morphine or other strong opioid drugs can give subjective relief for dyspnoea. Bronchodilators are only useful where reversible airways obstruction can be demonstrated. There is some anecdotal evidence to suggest that nebulized local anaesthetics may be useful in some patients. While having no specific effects on dyspnoea, reduction of the associated anxiety can be achieved using a small dose of benzodiazopines. Oxygen is often used but has only a placebo effect.

Cough. This can be a difficult symptom to control. Opioid drugs remain the mainstay in the form of codeine linctus or morphine elixir. Troublesome cough can be helped by nebulized local anaesthetics such as marcaine.

Headache. In patients with advanced breast cancer, headache may have many causes, and migraine and tension headaches are probably more common than is raised intracranial pressure associated with

cerebral metastases. If there are cerebral metastases they should be treated with a combination of cranial irradiation and dexamethasone 4 mg q.d.s.
Incontinence. There are a number of aids available to help with incontinence which reduces the distress that this causes.
Bone pain. Single fractions of radiotherapy to localized painful bony metastases are frequently effective. For more generalized bone pain, bisphosphonates can on occasion produce symptomatic relief.
Malodour. Odour from fungating tumours, septic bedsores, incontinence due to poor laundry are an embarrassment for patients. Odour from fungating tumours and infected bedsores can often be controlled by the application of antibiotics such as metronidazole gel.

General considerations

Hospice care

Doctors and nurses involved in palliative care are experts in alleviating symptoms of terminal illness. Providing the patient and general practitioner are agreeable, the hospice team should be contacted as early as possible, once it is appreciated that the patient is entering the terminal phase of their illness. It should be remembered that hospices can offer both out-patient as well as in-patient support.

Terminal care

For the majority of patients who die from metastastic breast cancer, death is not a sudden event. During this period the aim of management is to maintain the patient in a comfortable and peaceful condition. Although oral medication is possible in the initial phase, there comes a time when, because of impaired consciousness, oral medication is no longer possible and should be changed to either the rectal or parenteral route.

Maintaining patients at home

Early domestic support from district nursing services or local hospice nurses is invaluable. Patients and their relatives should be made fully aware of the resources which are available within and outwith the Health Service. These include Attendance Allowance (which can be made available speedily through the Special Rules) and various other allowances. Not enough consideration is given to the financial considerations; dying patients and their relatives should be put in touch with social workers and, where appropriate, local charities.

It should also be appreciated that the carers themselves suffer physical symptoms looking after patients in the terminal phase of their disease and may also require support.

8. Breast reconstruction

Reconstruction should be available to all women who need a mastectomy. Many will decline it, expressing the feeling that they have had or will have had enough surgery. Reconstruction may be either immediate or delayed. Immediate reconstruction is less time consuming for the patient (but not for the surgeon) but care has to be taken that an oncological operation is not jeopardized for a better cosmetic result. Some would say that one surgeon should not perform both operations although these comments are heard most often in the USA where two surgeons means more money!

The reconstruction can be carried out by either immediate placement of a prosthesis (usually in the subpectoral position), by placement of a tissue expander with subsequent stretching of skin and muscle and eventual replacement of the expander with a silicone prosthesis, or by a flap of muscle and skin. The two most common (myocutaneous) flaps used require movement of either part of the latissimus dorsi muscle (Fig. 8.1) with overlying skin or the lower abdominal fat and skin based on the rectus abdominis muscle (Transverse Rectus Abdominis Myocutaneous flap; TRAM) (Fig. 8.2). The latter may be carried out either as a rotational flap based on the superior epigastric artery or as a free flap using a microvascular anastamosis of the inferior epigastric vessels to the subscapular or thoracodorsal vessels.

TISSUE EXPANSION AND SILASTIC PROSTHESES

The scare about the safety of silastic implants has put some women off having this technique. Further studies are being undertaken in the USA but the licensing authority has allowed their use for reconstructive purposes. They are generally implanted after a period of tissue expansion. This involves placement of a plastic bag connected to a valve in a pocket created under the pectoralis major muscle. Saline is injected into the valve at weekly or fortnightly visits until the desired volume is achieved. It is usual to over-expand the reconstructed side and to keep it over-expanded for a period of time before substituting the definitive

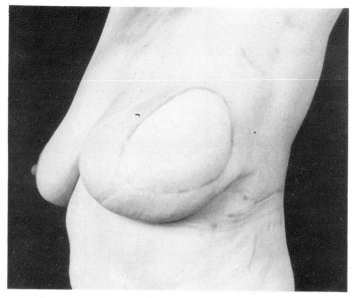

Fig. 8.1   Example of a latissimus dorsi rotational flap used for breast reconstruction.

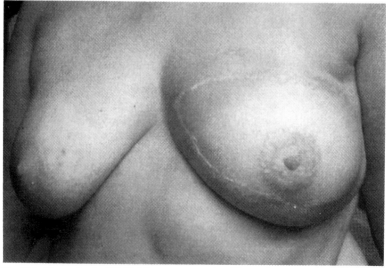

Fig. 8.2   Example of a TRAM flap reconstruction. Note subsequent nipple reconstruction.

prosthesis (Fig. 8.3). This often allows the capsule which forms around the bag to remain stretched and is said to reduce the rate of subsequent problems with capsular shrinkage.

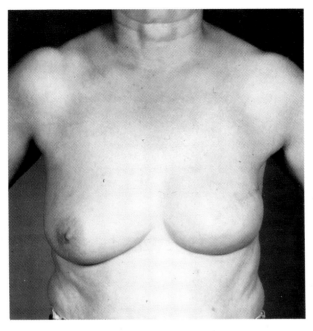

Fig. 8.3   Results of tissue expansion and then insertion of a prosthesis for breast reconstruction.

SUBCUTANEOUS MASTECTOMY

Patients with extensive DCIS or those having a prophylactic mastectomy may be offered a subcutaneous mastectomy with immediate placement of a subcutaneous prosthesis. This used to be unsatisfactory due to capsular contracture, which was easily seen when the prosthesis was just below the skin. This has been remedied to some extent by the use of textured surface or foam-covered prostheses. Others use a period of tissue expansion to try and achieve a better final cosmetic outcome. A newer technique reconstructing the breast with a de-epithelialized TRAM flap gives the most natural and aesthetically pleasing result. Subcutaneous mastectomy removes the majority of breast tissue but care has to be taken in planning incisions as there may be a problem in reaching all the breast tissue and, if the patient has already had a biopsy, areas of poor vascularity may result. A pad under the nipple is often left to preserve its blood supply but, even so, nipple necrosis is a potential complication. A biopsy of the pad under the nipple must be taken to ensure malignant cells are not present. Patients need to be aware that cancer can develop or recur under the nipple and that it may need resection.

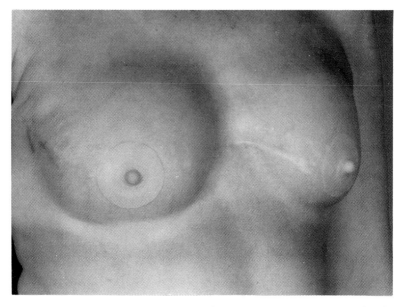

Fig. 8.5 A patient wearing her false nipple after breast reconstruction. (Reproduced with permission from Sainsbury et al 1991 Ann Roy Coll Surg Engl 73: 67–69.)

NIPPLE RECONSTRUCTION

The final touch after breast reconstruction. This can be carried out by a number of surgical techniques. Some require transplantation of darker skin (common donor sites being the skin behind the ear or from the labia) whereas others create a nipple using the skin of the breast and tattoo the skin to achieve a colour match. That there are so many techniques available is a reflection of how unsatisfactory many are in the long term.

Another technique is to use a stick on nipple which can be removed and worn by the patient at her will. The commercial varieties are unrealistic but it is possible to make a customized nipple by taking a plaster cast impression of the remaining side. A colour-matched silastic prosthesis is then made and is more realistic (Fig. 8.4) and carries greater patient acceptability (Fig. 8.5).

9. Clinical trials

The use of clinical trials has provided the information upon which a logical treatment for breast cancer can be based. The Lancet overview in early 1992 has confirmed that adjuvant chemotherapy provides major benefits for the premenopausal woman as does adjuvant tamoxifen for the postmenopausal woman. This review of 75 000 women from 133 randomized trials contained 31 000 recurrences and 24 000 deaths.

The history of trials can be divided into three eras. The early trials were basically of more versus less surgery and/or radiotherapy. Then came the trials of less surgery versus standard mastectomy. Finally the era of large trials on the role of chemotherapy and endocrine therapy came in.

The future of trials is uncertain — less that 2% of eligible patients are entered into a clinical trial (whether because of the clinicians disinclination or pressure of work or because the patient refuses randomization) despite the evidence that patients in trials receive better treatment and do better. They are expensive to run and require an input of time and effort that many clinicians find difficult to give.

The debate on how to achieve informed consent continues and a recent suggestion that women should be mobilized and trained to counsel patients is intriguing.

Psychology and breast disease

10. Psychological factors in patients with breast disease

George Masterton   Rhiannon Pugh

INTRODUCTION

It is convenient to consider psychological aspects under four main areas: antecedents; reactions to disease and treatment; factors in determining outcome; and counselling techniques and problems.

ANTECEDENTS

This issue is bedevilled by the variable and indeterminable lag between tumour onset and the presentation of the patient. Also, breast tumours may grow at varying and uneven rates and patients present at different stages, so distinguishing antecedents from reactions can prove difficult. Antecedents include mental illness, adverse life effects and cancer-prone personality (type C personality).

Mental illness

Depression as a potential precursor of cancer is an unresolved issue with evidence for a weak association in epidemiological research but conflicting findings in smaller studies of affected patients. In the case of breast cancer the likelihood of a patient having had a depressive illness treated during the preceding 5 years is no greater than for matched controls with benign breast disease.

Life events/stresses

Again, epidemiological studies tend to show a weak association between stressful events and the onset of cancer; but there is no evidence of an association between the diagnosis of breast cancer and preceding stressful life events of any severity, recent or remote, comparing affected women with matched women who have benign breast disease.

Cancer-prone personality

The picture is both different and fascinating as far as personality attributes predisposing to breast cancer are concerned, with a number of studies demonstrating fairly consistent differences in personality traits between women with breast cancer and those with benign or no breast disease. The main findings refer particularly to patients under 50 years of age and have also been reported less frequently in other female cancers.

The main personality traits, termed variously type C or cancer-proneness are low anxiousness, excessive suppression of anger and an enhanced tendency to avoid conflicts. Such women respond to stress by using a repressive coping style, i.e. they don't let their feelings show, a core facet which has been termed 'repressive defensiveness'. How this might be transduced into cancer-proneness is uncertain.

Managing the issue of control over cancer

The prospect that, for some patients, there are factors within their own character that may have contributed to the development of their breast tumour, can prove frightening or invigorating; and the doctor faced with a patient who is knowledgeable or curious about this must recognize this is a double-edged weapon that needs to be handled carefully.

Part of the polarization of views that sometimes arises between the patient and doctor occurs because doctors may either not fully appreciate the psychological attitudes of their patient or regard such ideas as competitive with their own: so instead of psychological interventions being regarded as complimentary they become alternative. There would be less rejection of orthodox medicine if these aspects and needs of the patient were taken into account.

REACTIONS

These include reactions to breast cancer, surgery and adjuvant treatments.

Breast cancer

Prevalence and morbidity

The prevalence of psychological disorders in the year following diagnosis and surgical treatment of breast cancer has consistently been reported around 30%, which is about three times what would be expected in the general population. Most patients carry a diagnosis of anxiety and/or depressive illness. These are typically mild disorders and, indeed, severe illnesses are only slightly more frequent than expected.

With such high levels of morbidity it may seem surprising that referral rates for psychological help are low; for instance the first 50 referrals from a breast cancer unit specialist liaison service were gleaned from around 3000 patients, i.e. only about 1.7% of all breast cancer patients were referred.

There are a number of explanations for the low levels of referral. One important reason may be the availability of appropriate local services. The discrepancy has, however, been mainly attributed to medical failings and, in particular, the failure of surgeons to enquire about the patient's emotional well-being or to recognize and treat their psychological symptoms, compounded by the reluctance of patients to disclose these aspects unless asked. On the other hand, it has been proposed that most of these cases reflect psychological pseudomorbidity rather than true illness and indeed even with a 1.7% referral rate the breast liaison service still reported half their patients had transient psychological reactions that required no more than brief counselling.

Adjustment reactions

For most women the threats, fears and losses associated with a breast lump, cancer and its treatment concern not just their health and survival, but their body image, sexuality and self-esteem, as well as their marriage, family life, work and social pursuits. These are not trivial matters and the emotional responses reflect the gravity of the situation.

Modulating thoughts, feelings and behaviours to cope with crisis is not a pathological process, rather it represents an adaptive response preparing the individual to adjust. Of course adjustment processes can become maladaptive either in degree, when an emotional illness requiring treatment develops, or in form, with abnormal coping responses such as extreme denial, deliberate self-harm, eating disorders, drug or alcohol abuse. However getting things out of proportion or going off the rails is usually something the patient, her family and/or her medical attendants recognize; and it is with the patient, supported and guided by others who know her, that the decision about the need for psychological intervention should rest, not with the presence of tears or a result on a psychiatric research scale.

Further, diagnosing mental disorder and prescribing treatment inappropriately is not harmless, especially if this is at variance with the patient's perspective. Adding the stigma of being a psychiatric patient to already distressing circumstances is one consequence; another is the generation of anxiety and misery through sentiments like 'something else is going wrong with me' and 'I ought to have been able to cope with this'.

The nurse counsellor

The great majority of the 30% of patients who are classified as suffering from psychiatric morbidity do not need, and would not benefit from psychiatric referral. They are suffering from understandable psychological reactions which usually respond well to brief intervention, often only one or two counselling sessions being required. This is best portrayed as part of the disease process and handled by the surgical team: this is where a nurse counsellor proves essential. This counsellor obviously requires psychological training, support and backup, and it is at this level that the specialist psychiatric service should operate, taking on those patients who are considered (particularly by the nurse counsellor) to be experiencing unduly severe or prolonged symptoms, as well as those who have coincidental psychiatric disorder or cerebral complications of their malignancy.

Surgical treatment

For many patients it is the treatment rather than the disease which turns out to be the more unpleasant and distressing aspect. In the quest for prolonging survival or cure doctors may underestimate the effects upon the patient of their work. In recent years particularly, increasing attention is being paid to the quality of life associated with cancer treatments.

Some of the findings concerning psychological responses associated with different surgical techniques may prove surprising. The most notable discovery is that emotional distress and psychological maladjustment is as frequent after lumpectomy as following mastectomy. The explanation appears to be that the removal of a breast leads to grieving for loss while conservation provokes mistrust about that breast with a fear cancer is still lurking and a mastectomy will prove inevitable.

Given the choice, two-thirds of women in one study opted for mastectomy rather than lumpectomy, essentially to get the business over and done with. However breast conservation (or immediate reconstruction) does appear to reduce psychiatric morbidity in women who are particularly concerned about their appearance at the time of surgery. The solution might be a 'horses for courses' approach so that when survival is not materially affected it is the patient's preference, if she has one, rather than surgical fashion that should be directive.

Where lumpectomy wins over mastectomy is in the area of satisfaction with body image. Mastectomized women tend to have lower self-esteem, greater social withdrawal and more frequent sexual dysfunction compared with women whose breast is retained. Of course breast reconstruction with a prosthetic implant following mastectomy offers a means of resolving these conflicting emotional reactions in that the fear of cancer is removed without destroying physical integrity to the same extent; and, certainly, this procedure restores a sense of satisfaction with body image although, with immediate reconstruction at least, beneficial effects upon emotional morbidity are not evident. It may be that improved technology and optimal timing of implant surgery will improve the psychological outcome, for these procedures still present problems in the frequency of surgical complications and subjective dissatisfaction with the cosmetic outcome.

About one in three women who enjoyed a satisfactory sexual relationship prior to surgery develop subsequent sexual problems, with loss of libido being most common. Sexual dysfunction is reported nine times more frequently among women with body image dissatisfaction compared with women who find their appearance acceptable.

Adjuvant treatment

The picture is clear with the adjuvant treatments of chemotherapy and radiotherapy. Postoperative radiotherapy can prove distressing for a few patients and is associated with more physical symptoms and social dysfunction during the course, but not with increased anxiety or depression.

Postoperative chemotherapy causes considerable psychological morbidity, especially with prolonged courses of treatment.

There has been little research upon the psychological effects of hormonal treatment. Tamoxifen does not appear to be associated with adverse psychological effects, but depression may be more frequent after oophorectomy. Finally, it should be borne in mind that none of these adjuvant therapies are associated with increased psychiatric morbidity once the course of treatment is completed.

VULNERABILITY FACTORS

What women are most at risk of developing psychiatric morbidity? Vulnerability factors include general factors which predispose women in middle life to emotional illness and factors specific to aspects of breast cancer and its treatment.

General factors include a previous history of psychiatric disorder and especially mood illness, an unsatisfactory or broken marriage, the lack of a confiding relationship, and major life stresses of an unwelcome nature.

Specific factors are notably the adjuvant treatments, chemotherapy and oophorectomy, where the additional risk is confined to the short term. Perhaps unexpectedly, in women with breast cancer being unmarried is protective.

FAMILY FACTORS

The patient's vulnerability can be increased by more subtle changes in the family dynamics than a cursory social history will reveal. It is established that the husbands of breast cancer patients suffer physical symptoms and psychological distress, and for some loving and otherwise confiding partners the way they cope is by denial or some other maladaptive mechanism. Maladjustment in the spouse can add to the patient's guilt and fear, especially in a previously sound relationship. In these circumstances sexual dysfunction is particularly common and distressing, and this compounds the problem.

The impact of cancer upon the rest of the family is a complex, important issue, yet in the case of breast cancer seems to have been relatively neglected in contrast to the efforts made to counsel the individual patient.

OUTCOME

The evidence that psychological factors contribute significantly to outcome, both in terms of mortality and relapse, is more compelling than for tumour genesis. Findings include mental illness, life events/stresses, personality and attitude/coping styles.

Mental illness

There is good evidence from a number of studies that women who are classified as a psychiatric case preoperatively have a better chance of disease-free survival at 5 and more years. Bearing in mind the distinction made between a case on a research scale and clinical practice, it is probably safer to interpret this finding as meaning that it is women who are distressed at the time of diagnosis or surgery who have a better prognosis, rather than those who are suffering from a true mental illness.

Life events/stresses

The role of severe life events in precipitating relapse in breast cancer patients is at present unsubstantiated.

Personality

There is good evidence that women with breast cancer who have type C personality traits or cope through repressive defensiveness are more likely to relapse compared with women who are not.

Attitudes/coping style

The best evidence that psychological features are independent mediators of disease-free survival comes from a study of only 57 patients first assessed in 1971 before biologically sophisticated measures such as hormone receptor status were widely available. Their method involved the patient's coping style being determined by the investigator upon verbatim statements and accompanying mood 3 months after simple mastectomy with attribution to one of four mutually exclusive categories — denial (apparent active rejection of any evidence about their diagnosis which might have been offered), fighting spirit (a highly optimistic attitude accompanied by a search for greater information about breast cancer), stoic acceptance (acknowledgement of the diagnosis without enquiry for further information unless new symptoms developed) and feelings of helplessness/hopelessness (complete engulfment by knowledge of the diagnosis).

5 years later patients who had been categorized as 'fighters' and 'deniers' were five to six times more likely to be surviving without recurrence compared with patients who had stoically accepted their lot or had decompensated into a helpless/hopeless state. This effect was maintained 10 and 15 years after assessment and could not be attributed to any crucial biological differences among the groups. Other studies from the UK, USA and Canada have since produced the same finding that deniers and/or fighters have a greater chance of disease-free survival when compared with other attitudes. The scale of this effect appears to be large, but its explanation remains obscure. Potential explanations involve relationships between psychological state and concentrations of immunoglobulins, natural killer cells, prolactin and tumour oestrogen and progesterone status.

BREAKING BAD NEWS

There is no good way to break bad news as, by definition, it is bad. What we need to think about then are ways to tell a woman that she has breast cancer which will make it easier for her to bear the news, to receive the information that she needs to know and to allow her to express her feelings and concerns.

The immediate impact

Upon learning that she has breast cancer a woman is liable to feel a number of complex emotions. She may feel shock, anxiety, anger, distress and sorrow. These will not be avoided no matter how the interview is carried out; however they may be mitigated if she is asked to bring along a close relative or friend, as this has been shown to reduce depression, anxiety and improve adjustment 1 year later. A friendly and unhurried interview with no interruptions will help. Allow the patient time to react to the news without rushing in prematurely with reassurance or advice. These are likely to be defensive manoeuvres on the part of the physician to distance himself from the patient's potentially strong emotions.

It is worthwhile trying to be guided by the patient who will let you know how much she wants to know by both verbal and non-verbal cues.

Improving the information giving process

Improved communication between doctors and their patients leads to better treatment compliance, improved trust and less likelihood of litigation. An essential aspect of communication is that of information giving.

Many doctors have difficulty with this part of their job. A study carried out in 1986 confirms this. 101 women with the diagnosis of early breast cancer were interviewed following the 'bad news' interview, and over half expressed dissatisfaction feeling that the information they had been given was inadequate. Surveys have shown that approximately half the information given to patients is forgotten and that approximately 50% of patients would like to ask questions but feel inhibited.

Ways to improve recall:

- Use the primary effect — patients remember information at the beginning of the interview better; therefore try to give the most important information then.
- Keep things simple — use shorter sentences, smaller words and avoid medical terminology.
- Use repetition — ask the patient to feedback what she has learned during the consultation.
- Use written information.
- Consider using other aids such as audiotapes of the consultation which the patient can then take home to replay.

Aiding the expression of emotions and concerns

As a profession we tend to greatly undervalue the benefits of listening to our patients and trying to understand them; this can be much more comforting than we often realize and it is worth trying not to succumb to the temptation to falsely reassure or give advice straightaway, as these measures can be a way of reducing our own discomfort and not that of the patient.

People choose their career's not only on reasons of which they are aware but also unconscious ones, often those going into Medicine have strong desires to cure others or at the least to make them feel better. This can create problems when dealing with cancer patients as doctors may feel conscious or unconscious anger, hopelessness or despair which can then lead to distancing, avoidance of emotional issues, false cheerfulness and optimism, concentration on purely physical aspects of the disease, etc. as a way of protecting himself/herself. This may leave the patient feeling bewildered, isolated and anxious.

To try to minimize these problems a practitioner needs to be aware that he may feel uncomfortable with cancer patients for a number of reasons but problems can be avoided with some degree of self-awareness. Practitioners working with cancer patients need support for themselves either formal or informal and should seek supervision from a mental health professional if they feel out of their depth. Once a patient feels confident that her doctor is able to tolerate her difficult emotions and is not going to be overwhelmed she will automatically feel more understood and will find this reassuring in itself.

COUNSELLING WOMEN WITH BREAST CANCER

It is easy to fall into the trap of imagining that we know the sort of feelings a woman might have on being treated for breast cancer; however, we cannot be sure and it is therefore very important to ascertain the meaning of both the disease itself and the treatment.

The disease

The term cancer has different meanings to different people depending on previous experience and fantasies. For example:

- Inevitable pain or death.
- Humiliation, shame, loss of dignity.
- Loss of control.

It is important to investigate ideas and beliefs about cancer and also to enquire about friends or relatives who have had cancer.

Women may feel that their bodies have betrayed them or are running amok, and may feel extremely concerned by any minor physical ailments worrying that these may herald a recurrence. Women can also feel their bodies to be extremely vulnerable, as if the boundaries between inside and outside have been weakened. This may affect their ability to partake in physical exercise, or even to venture into places where there may be accidental physical contact for example busy shopping centres.

The treatment

The breast is intimately bound up with femininity, sexuality and creativity. It may be that loss of, or perceived disfigurement of, the breast may be more distressing to a woman than actually having cancer itself. This is particularly likely if a woman's self-esteem is tied up with her appearance and sexual identity.

Mastectomy, oophorectomy and the use of anti-oestrogen drugs can all be perceived consciously or unconsciously as an attack on a woman's femininity. Depending on her previous experience this may lead to resentment and non-compliance with treatment. Another possible outcome is that she may no longer feel that she has 'permission' to be a woman which can lead to sexual difficulties. (In fact long-term sexual problems have been reported in 10–30% of women.) Gentle exploration of these issues may prove beneficial especially if a woman can be made aware of the reasons behind her reactions.

Chemotherapy and radiotherapy can cause a great deal of physical suffering and women often find themselves resenting the treatment but find it difficult to express angry feelings towards the doctors who are trying to help them. Patients also find it hard to tolerate the physical effects when there is no guarantee that the treatment will be effective. One particular side-effect which is distressing is the hair loss as some women complain that it grows back differently.

Problems which can arise during counselling

Things can go wrong if a patient uses defence mechanisms excessively or if something happens to cause relationship difficulties between patient and counsellor. This usually happens because of transference or countertransference reactions. These terms will be explained below.

Common psychological reaction to loss

Of course not all women with breast cancer will experience severe difficulties but some psychological adjustment is necessary.

Shock, anger, depression and acceptance all have their place when coming to terms with any loss and in fact are necessary. They will be recognizable to anyone working with bereaved patients or have been bereaved themselves. A patient does not work her way steadily through these feelings but will oscillate between them, gradually progressing towards acceptance. It is only if they are prolonged or very intense that we need to be worried.

Previous coping styles can provide us with some idea of how a woman is going to respond. Women who have been compulsively self reliant may find it difficult to relinquish control to doctors and also find fighting an invisible enemy a problem. Previously dependent patients may be easier to deal with as they find the regression to patient status easier, although there is a danger that they may become excessively dependent on those treating them.

Commonly used psychological defence mechanisms

Defence mechanisms are something that we all use and are unconscious 'mental tricks' to help us avoid anxiety and mental pain. There are many different types, but the following may be used by patients suffering from breast cancer and also dying patients:

- Denial — seeming not to be aware of diagnosis or prognosis; not a problem unless of such a degree that it prevents a patient from seeking proper treatment.
- Regression — reverting back to a more baby-like state; useful during acute illness but can be a problem during rehabilitation.
- Displacement — transferring feelings which belong to one person or situation onto another; e.g. anger with a doctor for late diagnosis may be inappropriately felt towards a spouse.
- Projection — feelings which really belong to oneself are projected on to others; e.g. a woman might unconsciously feel disgusted with her own body but projects that onto others ending up thinking that they find her disgusting.

Transference

This term means the development of feelings by the patient towards the therapist which really belong to important figures from the patient's past — usually parents. This usually aids treatment as it fosters trust and compliance. If however a patient has had a difficult relationship with her parents (possibly abusive) then she will re-enact this with her doctor, complaining that he/she is cold, uncaring, cruel or however it was that she experienced them. Recognizing this and, if necessary, exploring these feelings with the patient can prevent serious breakdown in communications.

Countertransference

This refers to those feelings that a patient stirs up in her therapist. Modern psychotherapists believe that these can be a form of unconscious communication. For example a doctor may feel unaccountably despairing or overwhelmed when faced with a particular patient. If these are unusual feelings for him/her it is possible that a woman is communicating her own feelings about having cancer. Alternatively a therapist may feel unreasonably angry or irritable. Sensitive therapists can use these feelings to explore further how their patients really feel and if they show that they can tolerate them this does bring great feelings of relief.

Of course feelings can also originate in the therapist himself as he has a wealth of life experiences behind him and has built up his own defences and ways of dealing with situations. If the feelings engendered by a patient within the therapist are particularly uncomfortable, strong or uncharacteristic they should be considered as a potential communication of how the patient is feeling.

Psychotherapy with the dying patient

When a patient is dying the defence mechanisms of denial and regression are commonly brought into play and are extremely effective in aiding the patient to make the most of the end of her life and to die peacefully. Women who are experiencing excessive anxiety or depression may benefit from a bolstering of these defences.

This can be brought about by the use of transference; if a patient feels that someone is concerned and caring for them in a maternal way they feel protected and are able to regress which can reinforce denial. Trust in the therapist is essential. The therapist must tell the truth to any questions the patient asks, should be consistent in his/her approach to the patient and should be reliable. These therapist characteristics will foster positive feelings in the patient which will resemble previous infantile feelings towards her mother.

This is a time when patients really need to feel that they are being listened to, so it is better not to be in a hurry to 'do' something. Most anxieties about dying are not existential in nature but are to do with the manner of dying. Reassurance about pain relief and alleviation of other physical symptoms can be immensely comforting.

Monitoring one's own feelings again can be a useful guide to a patient's state of mind. Working with the dying can be enormously stressful because it can stir up feelings and fantasies that the therapist has about his own mortality and any previous personal experience of death. We do build up our own defence mechanisms to help us deal with this, but sometimes if they become too effective the therapist will seem cold and remote. Alternatively the therapist may become over-identified with the patient recognizing aspects of himself in them, in this case the patient may complain that the therapist was intrusive and had lost his objectivity. Obviously different patients will stir up different feelings in therapists but if a response has become habitual it may be worth looking more closely at our own feelings in case our own defences are getting in the way.

Further reading

Bland KI, Copeland EM 1991 The breast. Comprehensive management of benign and malignant diseases. WB Saunders, Philadelphia

Bostwick J III 1990 Plastic and reconstructive breast surgery. Quality Medical Publications, St Louis, Missouri

de Moulin D 1989 A short history of breast cancer. Kluwer Academic Publishers, Dordrecht, Germany

Dixon JM 1992 Breast surgery in Taylor EW (ed.) Infection in surgical practice. Oxford University Press, Oxford

Dixon JM 1993 Breast conservation surgery in Taylor I, Johnson CD (eds) Recent advances in surgery 16. Churchill Livingstone, Edinburgh

Fallowfield LJ, Baum M 1984 Psychological welfare of patients with breast cancer. J R Soc Med 82: 4–5

Forrest P 1990 Breast cancer: the decision to screen. Nuffield Provincial Hospital Trust, London

Greer HS, Morris T, Pettingale KW 1979 Psychological response to breast cancer: effect on treatment. Lancet ii: 785–787

Hughes LE 1989 Progress symposium – Benign breast disorders: fibrocystic disease? or non disease? or ANDI. World J Surg 13: 667–764

Hughes LE, Mansel RE, Webster DJT 1989 Benign disorders and diseases of the breast. Balliere Tindall, London

Ley P 1988 Communicating with patients. Croom Helm, London

Page DL, Anderson TJ 1988 Diagnostic histopathology of the breast. Churchill Livingstone, Edinburgh

Powles TJ, Smith IE 1991 Medical management of breast cancer. Martin Dunitz, London

Ramirez A 1984 Liason psychiatry in a breast cancer unit. J R Soc Med 82: 15–17

Smallwood JA, Taylor I 1990 Benign breast disease. Edward Arnold, London

Stewart HJ, Anderson TJ, Forrest APM 1991 Breast disease: new approaches. Br Med Bull 47: 251–522

Index